MIND YOUR BREATHING

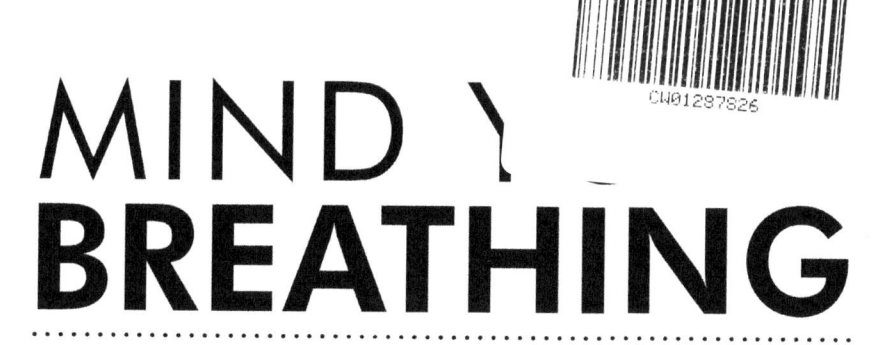

THE YOGI'S HANDBOOK WITH
37 PRANAYAMA EXERCISES

SUNDAR
BALASUBRAMANIAN
PH.D, C-IAYT

notionpress.com

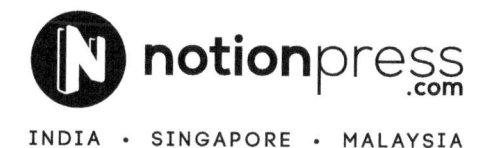

INDIA · SINGAPORE · MALAYSIA

Notion Press

Old No. 38, New No. 6
McNichols Road, Chetpet
Chennai - 600 031

First Published by Notion Press 2019
Copyright © Sundar Balasubramanian 2019
All Rights Reserved.

ISBN 978-1-68466-842-7

This book has been published with all efforts taken to make the material error-free after the consent of the author. However, the author and the publisher do not assume and hereby disclaim any liability to any party for any loss, damage, or disruption caused by errors or omissions, whether such errors or omissions result from negligence, accident, or any other cause.

While every effort has been made to avoid any mistake or omission, this publication is being sold on the condition and understanding that neither the author nor the publishers or printers would be liable in any manner to any person by reason of any mistake or omission in this publication or for any action taken or omitted to be taken or advice rendered or accepted on the basis of this work. For any defect in printing or binding the publishers will be liable only to replace the defective copy by another copy of this work then available.

Contents

Foreword 9

Preface 15

Acknowledgments 19

Introduction 21

General Considerations for the Pranayama Exercises 29

1. Dheerga Swasam (Deep Breathing) 33
2. Pranava Pranayama (Om Chanting) 36
3. Anuloma Viloma Pranayama (Alternate Nostril Breathing) 39
4. Viloma Pranayama (Stepped Alternate Nostril Breathing) 41
5. Chandra Nadi Pranayama (Left Nostril Breathing) 45
6. Surya Nadi Pranayama (Right Nostril Breathing) 47
7. Thirumoolar Pranayama (TMP) 50
8. Kukriya Pranayama (Panting Breathing) 53
9. Kapalabhati (Shining Skull) 56
10. Bhastrika (Bellows of Breath) 59

11. Agnisara Kriya (Fire Rising) 62

12. Sudharsana Chakra Kriya (Solar Plexus Exercise) 64

13. Thee Moochu (Breath of Fire) 67

14. Ujjayi (Ocean Sound Breathing) 70

15. Bhramari (Humming Bee Breathing) 73

16. Savithri Pranayama (Rectangular Breathing) 76

17. Sama Vritti (Balanced Breathing) 79

18. Vishama Vritti (1:2 Breathing) 81

19. Nan Madi Moochu (Four Part Breathing) 83

20. Padi Moochu (Multistep Breathing) 85

21. Pongu Moochu (Fountain Breathing) 87

22. Ahavoli Moochu (Illuminating Heart Breathing) 90

23. Pidari Marga Moochu (Back Route Breathing) 94

24. Puyal Moochu (Storm Breathing) 97

25. Mandhira Moochu (Mantra Breathing) 100

26. Sheetali Pranayama (Rolling Tongue Breathing) 104

27. Sheetkari Pranayama (Smiling Breathing) 107

28. Sithan Pokku Moochu (Sithar's Way Breathing) 110

29. Vizhi Nokku Moochu (Gaze-Controlled Breathing) 114

30. Sadhura Moochu (Square Breathing) 117

31. Sundara Chakra Pranayama 119

32. Karuvur Sithar Pranayama 129

33. Karai Moochu (Crying Breathing) 133

34. Kottavi Moochu (Yawning Breathing) 137

35. Thantha Moochu (Tooth Breathing) 141

36. Kireeda Moochu (Crown Chakra Churn Pranayama) 144

37. 166 Mathirai Moochu (166 Count Breathing) 147

Further Learning *151*

Backword *153*

Foreword

Having been a medical researcher for many years, it is always a joy to meet a colleague in the field. Sundar and I met in 2013 at Yogaville, VA when he attended Yoga of the Heart (a certification to adapt the sacred practices of Yoga for students with cardiac disease and cancer). Meeting him, I had a more complete feeling than what I often experience with other researchers. At the time, I attributed it to the fact that Sundar has been doing research in the rarefied field of Yogic practices for the past several years, while having academic roots from a traditional learning background. He shares what his research has yielded about the subtlety of Pranayama practices for patients' well being, and education.

I felt an immediate sense of kindness and a desire to share the data that he formulated. He seemed incapable of exaggerating the findings to make himself seem important; rather, he wanted to make it available to enhance other people's lives. Because his research involves ancient practices rather than a pill or gadget, the retail portion was exempt. He had a sparkle in his eye and a sense of peace that can only come from many years of dedicated spiritual practice. It was soon obvious that this was not an ordinary researcher, or ordinary research. It does not surprise me at all that the talk he offered as a part of the TEDx series, is one of the most highly viewed talks on Pranayama!

It is now fashionable to investigate the practices and effects of Yoga from a modern, scientific perspective. Yoga, being more than 5000 years old, can easily hold its own in any category from anecdotal evidence alone.

The practices that evolved over the millennia were not necessarily meant as a curative agent for the ills of the body; rather, they were touted as tools for total transformation. Medical science as we know it emerged just a few hundred years ago, and in some cases, exhibits strong enthusiasm to prove and validate the ancient practices.

The body, mind, emotions and spirit, when given the essential ingredients needed to come into balance, become whole. Our life, as well as the health of the body, becomes fit and able to function optimally for many years. The challenge is to determine which practices initiate the healing and balance of our being. There is also a need to modify existing methods for a variety of practitioners at all levels.

There were times when life was simpler, and discernment was a bit more simple too. With our busyness and fascination with the external, the more essential aspects are often forgotten. The scientific offerings can help us to discern which practices enhance, and even correct, imbalances in body, mind, and energy. It seems that when our focus went elsewhere, modern science stepped in with some answers.

Western science is still trying to discover what yogis have known for thousands of years, that the body, mind, and spirit are not separate. Even speaking about the body-mind connection is not entirely correct. It is not possible to separate them, except in theory.

In this landmark book, The Pranayama Handbook, we are offered practices that heighten our spiritual awareness, as well as fill in a large gap in the scientific field. There are very few modern resources to help us learn Pranayama techniques today, so this book is very timely.

Many of the sacred techniques are still held hostage by languages unfamiliar to many of us wanting to learn these life-changing practices. There has been a real need to translate this vital information from the Tamil literature to English, and thanks to Sundar, it has been done. This book contains step-by-step instructions for 37 traditional, modified, and completely new Pranayama exercises. Most were formulated and revealed during Sundar's personal longtime practice, in tandem with his scientific knowledge.

As we are told, and some of us experience, Pranayama is one of the great practices in the system of Hatha Yoga where the body, mind, and breath, all function together.

Many practitioners of Asana often disregard Pranayama completely or incorporate it as an adjunct to Asana. Today, there are many different styles and adaptations of Asana, yet there is no such innovation in the area of Pranayama.

Asana benefits and effects encourage the use of Pranayama to move oxygen through the system with each squeeze, bend, and stretch of the body. Through this process of re-oxygenation, the by-product of carbon dioxide, which has caused a toxic buildup, is eliminated. Others hail Pranayama for its use in calming the mind before entering a state of meditation, stilling the energy and thereby quieting the mind. Both of these assertions are correct. It is in the limitation of this practice that we have to pay close attention. We need to call to memory that Prana is the vital energy that permeates our entire being, and is,therefore, virtually everywhere. It can be used to assist in Asana and as a prelude for meditation. However, Pranayama of its own accord also holds infinite possibilities.

The Yoga Sutras of Patanjali, express it like this:

II.49 The universal life force (prana) is enhanced and guided through the harmonious rhythm of the breath (Pranayama).

II.50 The movement of the life force is influenced by inhalation, exhalation and sustained breath.

II.51 A balanced rhythmical pattern steadies the mind and emotions causing the breath to become motionless.

II. 52 As a result, the veils over the inner light are lifted.

II.53 The vista of higher consciousness is revealed.

Explained in 5 successive sutras, when the breathing pattern is balanced, it unlocks the bridge between the body and mind. We know that movements in our body affect our breathing. When we suddenly run or quicken our pace, the oxygen and energy requirements go up, and we breathe faster. When we slow down, our breath follows.

The opposite is also true; as our breathing patterns change, our body is also affected. If we are breathing shallowly, we may feel tired; a deep breath can fill us with vital energy, making us more alert.

The pattern of breath also directly affects the mind. It becomes a great aid for calming, as well as energizing the mind. Awareness of the breath can bring vitality and enjoyment to each moment of life. By exhaling slowly, we immediately release any strain or stress that has crept into our body or mind. Our breath becomes a great barometer for relaxation and stress. As we align our energies in this way, through regulation of the breath, we maintain calm through the ordinary emotional roller-coaster rides we encounter each day. We find that when we are upset, everything around us reflects the same disturbance as if it is somehow contagious. When tranquility prevails, it magnetizes everything with the same sense of calmness. In its simplest form, we get calm. In its most rarefied form, it changes the cells and we are healed. Can Pranayama actually do this? It seems the answer from Sundar's research findings is a resolute YES!

I and others who diligently partake in these timeless practices feel deep gratitude to Sundar for the release of this book at this crucial time. We now have in our hands a key to balance and ultimate wholeness, which we are finding out scientifically leads to healing.

Mind Your Breathing: The Yogi's Handbook with 37 Pranayama Exercises is a precious gift for us all!

– **Nischala Joy Devi**

Spiritual Teacher and Author, The Healing Path of Yoga and The Secret Power of Yoga, A Woman's Guide to the Heart and Spirit of the Yoga Sutras.

Buckingham, VA
January 29, 2019

Preface

It has been a little over two years since my first book *PranaScience: Decoding Yoga Breathing* was published. In the interim I have traveled significantly within the US, India, and Canada, giving workshops, teacher training, and speeches. The venues include Yoga studios, academic institutions, Yoga festivals, patient education conferences, and scientific meetings. Simultaneously there are several publications, interviews, and articles published on my research. With the grace of my Gurus, I have been able to do a good job disseminating whatever little I have learned from the Siddhars. I am very happy to see the excitement that the topic of my research brings among the audience based on the feedback. At the end of every meeting, I am filled with joy, hope, peace, satisfaction, and excitement that the time for Pranayama research has come.

One lacuna I see in this area is that there are no technical handbooks for Pranayama. Of course, there are numerous videos online, released by wonderful people who love sharing their knowledge. However, there are only a handful of written books on Pranayama techniques, and those too are limited by the number of exercises that they cover. My first thought was to write a book on how to do each exercise. I originally thought that I should go deep into every exercise and explain all the research if any done on those exercises, bringing related wisdom from the Siddha literature to the practice. However, in the meantime the need for a basic how to book, irrespective of whether more information on the basis of the research is available or not, dominated my preference. So I started putting together this book. Once I started writing, I began to develop new exercises as well. For instance, one early morning, when I was at the parking lot waiting for my shuttle bus to work, I saw the twinkling stars and took a deep breath. The songs that I had just heard in the car were still reverberating in my ears "Unaithinam thozhudhilan – Arunagirinathar" (உனைத் தினம் தொழுதிலன் - அருணகிரிநாதர்). This song talks about the deficiencies that a person has, including not thinking about the Divine, and about ways of reaching the oneness. This type of feeling had also been there in other literary works I had been reading and listening to within those past few days. They include:

"நானே பொய், என் நெஞ்சும் பொய்,

என் அன்பும் பொய், ஆனால் வினையேன்

அழுதால் உன்னைப் பெறலாமே"

— மாணிக்கவாசகர்

("Naane poy, en nenjum poy, en anbum poy, aanaal vinayen azhudhaal unnai peralaame" – Manickavasakar)

I am falsehood

My heart is a myth

My love is a deceit

But if I cry I can get you (Lord)

– Manickavasakar in Thiruvasakam

This is exactly the same feeling I got when I went to the church where they said the prayer about acknowledging our sins and praying for mercy. When we cry, when we acknowledge our deficiencies, that is the beginning of our travel towards the inner space. All these thoughts and the twinkling stars, and the nice morning breeze made me start sobbing.

The deep breath that I was taking became a stepwise sobbing, that sounded like a stepped Ujjayi. I discovered that this type of breathing was similar to crying. I did a couple of rounds of that exercise and found that it stimulated Suzhumunai (Sushumna) Nadi. My eyes were filled with tears. I felt that my heart was overflowing. When I got onto the bus I found that everyone on the bus was a part of myself. I realized that crying was an important physiological function that prepares us for a healing process, and more acceptance of the circumstances and events in our lives. When I did more research into the underpinnings of crying, and its effect on our mental and physical systems, I was convinced that we should cry more than just a few times a month, or that we should at least mimic crying so we can address some of the unattended or avoided emotions and process them. This is how I got into the Karai Pranayama explained in this book. There are several new exercises in this book, which arose similarly, by watching myself and experimenting with the breathing. I also believe that there is a component of grace from the Gurus in this process. Certain exercises were developed long ago and taught in several workshops before, for instance, the Sundara Chakkara Pranayama.

This book is a tool to learn the techniques and to understand the basis to some extent. For some exercises, I have given the possible mechanism, but that is not the case for several other exercises. I am sure that each exercise will open up numerous possibilities for several new practices within the Pranayama communities. Similar to numerous dancing movements, Yoga Asana postures, and songs, there will be numerous Pranayama methods and sequences, and each one will serve somebody. This book uses Moochu (means breathing in the Tamil language) as the word equivalent to Pranayama, the way I was taught. There are no strict rules to breathe! You breathe the way your mind and body ask you to breathe. When you listen, the breath works with you. It takes you to a state of higher consciousness and better health. I am not providing the exact quantities of spices, time to boil or quantity to make when it comes to your soup. I am only providing a generic recipe for the dish.

You have to make your own. Do not try to follow this book verbatim; use your inner Guru as your companion. You will be amazed, just I have been, with how many doors these exercises can open up within you—just through breathing.

Happy breathing!

Acknowledgments

First and foremost I would like to thank all my teachers for being the guides and the inspiration for these exercises. Some of the exercises were taught to me directly from my Gurus and some of them were given to me through their blessings. Without their blessings, this book would not have been a possibility. At the time of finishing this book, a new chapter in my life was taking shape, in the form of a project called Thirumoolar Tamil Chair. This project is energized by the support of the Tamil Chair Inc., the organization which installed the Harvard Tamil Chair. I thank all the individuals from Tamil Chair Inc, particularly – Dr. Sornam Sankar, Dr. Vijay Janakiraman, Dr. Sundaresan Sambandam, Dr. Bala Swaminathan, Mr. Kumar Kumarappan, Mrs. Vaidehi Herbert, and Mr. Appadurai Muttulingam that support this endowed chair project—a much-needed one for the advancement of Pranayama research. Organizations such as Tamil Sangams, Indian associations, temples, churches, academic institutions and Yoga studios, and individuals from across the globe support me for the Thirumoolar Tamil Chair project. This encouragement gave me the necessary momentum to finish this book, and to use it as a tool for fundraising. Part of the proceeds from this book will go to the establishment of Thirumoolar Tamil Chair.

Whenever I come up with a new technique I test it on myself several times, and then try it on my most adorable experimental models, my fellow practitioners! Most likely they are the ones that would be attending the workshop in the following week or the ones at the Holy Cow Yoga Center where I teach a weekly Pranayama class. Their feedback is very valuable in reassuring me that I am going on the right path. In fact, the questions raised by fellow practitioners on the availability of learning materials was the initiator to work on this book. I thank them all, including the hardworking Karma Yogis who organized these workshops and events.

When I wanted to include pictures in this book to explain the postures, and discussed this with Balaji Parthasarathi, he met with me on the same day. He did a great job on the pictures. Josh Goodwin is another wonderful soul who provided pictures for this book, which were taken during the video recording of the Gentle Yoga Yogic Breathing video lessons that I produced for my research studies. I thank both of them for making the best out of my poses!

As always my family and friends have been a great support for me to write this book. Constant interaction with many of them and my mentors helps me walk on the chosen path. Janaki and the kids Masilan, Nelli and Vetri were very patient with me for not being with them on many of the weekends, school events, and family movie nights in the living room. My sincere thanks to Carley Juel Stanley, an inspiring soul working on the public relations of the PranaScience Institute, for reading this book and providing valuable edits that have greatly improved the readability of the book.

My first book was published by Notion Press, and I like how they handle the production, marketing, and customer care. Anisha has done a great job on the illustrations, and Thaatcher was so helpful in the overall production. So I decided to stick with them for this book as well. I thank the Notion Press team for bringing out this book in the way I imagined.

Introduction

மெய்ப்பொருள் காண்பது அறிவு

- திருக்குறள்

The purpose of knowledge is to find the truth

– Thirukkural

In the journey of Yoga, Pranayama is an important hub. It is also a busy hub. There are people who have marked this hub as their destination. For some, it is a transit. Some may linger for quite some time, some run through quickly. Some miss their next carrier and have to wait longer. Some enjoy the experience here, and some want to move away quickly. Several originations from the East and West have Pranayama as their transit. It does not matter which particular religion, or era, or when they used Pranayama as a tool for spiritual seeking. It might not have been called Pranayama, but it involves breathing. It involves the connectivity that the breath brings between the mind and body. Pranayama belongs to everyone who uses breathing as a key to open the doors to higher spiritual experiences. It could be a singer from Thanjavur who uses the breathing techniques to bring out the extraordinary notes or a marathon runner in Boston who uses efficient breathing techniques to accomplish their goal. Pranayama is a collection of regulated breathing practices that can potentially impact the mind and body. These exercises were developed, organized and disseminated by seekers from various traditions including the saints from ancient India that in Tamil called the Siddhars (or Sithars). They have a prominent role in the development of Pranayama, as well as in other Yoga techniques. The Sithars are said to have learned the techniques from Nandhi, sometimes also referred to as Lord Siva, in a specific academic lineage that started from four of the Janaka Saints: Sivayoga Mamuni, Patanjali, Vyakramar, and Thirumoolar. From these eight Saints subsequent lineages branched out, and the eighteen Sithars who made significant contributions to the understanding of Siddhanta, Vedhanta, and Yoga philosophies are considered unique in their expressive, cryptic and enriched poems. Several of the Sithar poems are still in palm leaf manuscript forms, or in secluded pockets of the knowledge base, or in the first printed editions of certain religious organizations (called Aadheenams), or only in the Tamil language. This makes it difficult to understand and interpret the breadth and depth of the wisdom within that philosophical system. However, several Pranayama techniques from the Sithar traditions have made it into public use today. At least some of the widely used Pranayama techniques, for example, the Anuloma Viloma have been researched using modern biological tools so the biological mechanism is getting clear. This introduction summarizes some of the key aspects of Pranayama in order to provide a brief theoretical background before going into the actual techniques.

Mind and Body

The concept of Panjakottam (Panjakosha) explains our organization into body, breath, mind, wisdom, and bliss sheaths. As one can see, the breath sheath or the Pranamaya Kottam is in between the body on the outside and the mind on the inside. Therefore it is said to be the bridge connecting the two. Prana maya kottam is also called the vital energy sheath a the Prana is the flow of vital energy. Several poems from Sithar tradition strongly indicate that the breath is the horse that needs to be tamed; so one has to master it in order to travel deep into one's own self. The breath that is unattended will leave the master. Fortunately, we have this wonderful tool called the body that has a lot of true natural potential residing within it. When one can realize this potential within themselves, they will have so much to offer to the world. This is the way of liberation, or mukti, and the attainment of one's life goals. Therefore it is important to take care of the body; especially with the tool that has the potential to benefit both the mind and the body, Pranayama.

Breathing is an autonomic nervous system function; it occurs whether we watch it or not. We breathe about fifteen times each minute (21,600 times a day). However, controlling the breathing rate, or retention, or using the breathing as a way to focus on one thing has been an effective way to reap benefits for the mind and the body. It also provides an opportunity for going deeper into the Panjakottam, to transcend into deeper spaces like the bliss sheath and to reach ultimate nirvana or enlightenment or Samadhi, where we become one with the nature. Whatever may be the goal for an individual, perhaps it is just doing the daily chores, performing routine duties, or stimulating the intellectual potentials, or going on the path of higher consciousness, spirituality, or devotion, everyone can use Pranayama techniques. Pranayama can affect the physical and emotional systems, which is explained in the subsequent sections below.

Physical and Emotional Wellbeing: Overall physical system: Pranayama, since it involves voluntary control of breathing, can directly influence respiration and circulation primarily. By altering the number of breaths, the intensity with which the respiration goes on, or the involvement of breath retention if any, Pranayama can improve the functions of the lungs. There are studies showing an improvement in lung functions after only a few weeks of practicing Pranayama. Results include improved attention span, reduction in heart rate, normalization of blood pressure, reduction in reaction time to visual and auditory cues, and improved heart rate variability. Oxygen consumption changes with regard to the type of Pranayama, and the length of the exercise time.

Nervous system: What goes on in the brain during Pranayama practice is very interesting. Several studies show how Pranayama can change brain waves, essentially the electric current that a group of nerve cells generates when working together. There are specific frequencies that define each wave, and they can be measured by electrodes placed on the scalp or within the brain itself. These waves work together like a symphony orchestra to alter specific functions, for instance, the activation of theta waves by the feeling of fear can be a potential communication between the amygdala and the hippocampus. This particular wave can be created by the Bhramari breathing for instance. This creates a possibility that the practice of Bhramari would provide factors that could make the otherwise fearful situations less fearful. Interestingly Bhramari could produce other types of waves too. It requires more rigorous studies.

Pranayama also can improve volumes of gray matter, as well as hippocampus size. Slow breathing has been shown to induce higher order brain functions including attention and memory through the regulation of locus coeruleus. Also, the involvement of olfactory lobes that are located in the upper respiratory tract, having a direct connection with the brain through the olfactory neurons, can function as a potential communicator to the brain about the external environment including temperature, humidity, scent, and the quality of breathing frequency. Thus, the respiratory system is an essential conduit between the environmental cues and the corresponding response by the brain. Research from my laboratory established for the first time that breathing regulation could stimulate changes in salivary biomarkers that have potential clinical applications. Activation of the parasympathetic nervous system, the vagal nerve stimulation, overall relaxation, and the inhibition of flight or fight response (sympathetic dominance) are the major outcomes of some of the Pranayama techniques. This aids in restorative and healing processes within both the physical and emotional systems.

Emotional regulation: Because of the strong impact by the breathing on the emotional regulating machinery of the brain, namely the limbic system, Pranayama is able to alter our perceptions. Slow breathing exercises can have a calming effect, whereas fast breathing exercises, when done vigorously, can have an activating effect on the body. Physiological and psychological stressors could have an adverse effect during chronic uncontrolled stimulation of stress responses. In these cases, the use of Pranayama could be beneficial to regulate the stress response elements.

Molecular level changes: Studies, including those from our laboratory, indicate that Pranayama could alter molecular makeup of the body. Reduction in stress hormone levels and specific biomarkers of metabolic alterations have been shown. We have shown the induction of salivary biomarkers, where saliva is considered an important fluid stimulated with the practice of Yoga. These biomarkers include nerve growth factor (NGF), immune response factors, tumor suppressors, pain and inflammatory biomarkers, blood pressure modifying enzymes, and molecules with potential regenerative capacities. Our studies form the first set of evidence showing the link between Pranayama, saliva, and molecular markers, and they have strong implications in the prevention and management of various illnesses. Being a systemic practice, Pranayama could stimulate changes in biomarkers all over the body via molecular transport, gene expression, enzyme activation, and other cellular signaling pathways. These are some of the novel concepts for future medical research.

Clinical applications: Owing to the above effects on the physical and emotional systems, Pranayama has the potential to be used in several psychosomatic disorders. Several studies, including our own, have shown that Pranayama has the potential to be useful in addressing some of the emotional aspects of chronic illnesses including anxiety and depression associated with cancer. Pranayama could improve mood, relaxation, and reduce fatigue, pain, and sleeplessness. Patients with diabetes and hypertension have shown better outcomes after Pranayama practice. Our identification of NGF and other neurotrophins after Pranayama provides the possibility that these techniques could be useful in delaying the progression of neurodegenerative diseases such as Alzheimer's and

Parkinson's disease, as well as being useful in recovery from stroke and other cardio/cerebrovascular diseases. Post-traumatic stress (PTS) is another major area where Pranayama is helpful as the PTS arises in the same neurocognitive systems that Pranayama targets. This provides a window of opportunity to avoid numerous suicides of veterans – almost 20 lives lost just in the US every day. PTS is not just a case of war veterans; it also affects millions of survivors, and victims of wars, violence, and other forms of trauma. Broad molecular and systemic effects elicited by Pranayama make this an attractive and cost-effective way of managing several illnesses making it an important adjunct practice to be used in the future among healthcare systems worldwide.

Pranayama Methods: Based on the Yoga literature from the ancient texts within the Sithar and other Indian contexts, there could be at least fifty different exercises. However, in the popular Yoga traditions throughout the world, only a handful of them are taught and practiced because many other techniques are not explained so far, or they have been buried deep within systems that are not yet popularized, for instance, the Siddha system. The practice of Pranayama can include the regulation of breathing (direct techniques), singing and chanting (indirect techniques), and other activity related techniques, for instance, how to regulate breathing during physical work, running and swimming, etc. There are some natural regulations of breathing occurring in our daily life, for example, yawning and sighing, that are stimulated based on the physical and emotional status. Cultural systems have incorporated specific ways of indirectly incorporating breathing regulation to address the potential development of adverse effects associated with the activity. For instance, postpartum depression could be managed by breathing techniques indirectly employed by singing a lullaby. Singing during joy, death, hard labor, and boredom is a way to process emotions through breathing alterations so they do not cause any long term damage to one's existence. As the chaotic theory is recognized to play a role in how the immune system functions, like the snowball effect, where small things accumulate over time to produce a large effect, the opposite could be true for causing greater goodness with small goodness created through a single good breath with mindfulness. While Pranayama, similar to the broad practice of Yoga, is misunderstood in some sectors as a religious practice, every culture, religious practice, or cultural sector has its own direct or indirect ways of practicing Pranayama. The name of the practice could be different, just like the religions have different names for one God, but the practice is to eventually regulate one thing, the breathing, and its effects are significant on the mind and body.

General Considerations for the Pranayama Exercises

Before learning the exercises, it is important to consider some of the common rules and safety aspects of Pranayama practice.

Food

Food is a necessary part of our lives. Maintaining healthy eating habits is important to our overall well-being. Moderation in what we eat and how much we eat is vital. Too much food will hamper breathing. Indigestion, gas, and heartburn are some of the inconveniences that can interfere with proper Pranayama practice. If we eat the right amount required for our body after the previous meal has been completely digested then there is no need for any medicine, according to Thirukkural. You do not have to be a vegetarian to regulate your breathing and do not let that be a factor to postpone your Pranayama. Drink adequate fluid throughout the day but try not to consume an excessive amount prior to your practice.

Timings

Any time is a good time to practice mindful breathing! You can watch your breathing, regulate it, and gain mastery over your Prana at any given time. However, there are certain times that would be good for certain fast breathing exercises or for regular practice. Early mornings, noon, and evening are good times suggested by Thirumoolar because each one will have an effect on our specific Vatha (noon), Pitha (morning), Kapa (evening) systems. Practicing three times can be a good way to balance the body. Having a routine might be helpful. Come up with your own creative ways to incorporate some breathing exercises during your day-to-day activities. For example, I use chanting, singing, and humming as a way of practicing Pranayama while driving. You can do a brief practice ahead of every meal or snack or drink. Do not practice fast breathing exercises immediately after a meal. Wait at least a few hours or until the food is digested. After a good one hour Pranayama session, wait at least 10–20 minutes to take your meal. This will help the factors that were stimulated with the Pranayama practice to get distributed within the body before you eat. If you are bored in a waiting room, or airport lounge, do not look at screens; close your eyes and look at your breathing. Nothing can make your time fly faster than breathing! Reserve a few minutes for a bedtime Pranayama. Before going to bed, take a few minutes to slow down the breathing, watch it, and do some gentle breathing exercises so you can have a nice deep sleep.

Postures and Locations

Sitting up crossed legged (Sukhasana), lotus pose (Padmasana) or Vajrasana are good postures in general for Pranayama. It can also be practiced while sitting in a chair upright or reclined, depending upon the exercise and the physical condition of the practitioner. Certain exercises can be done while lying down on a bed or while walking. The practice of Yoga postures (Asanas) is a good time to understand the flow of breath, and several breathing exercises could be creatively integrated into the Asana practice. Make sure the location where you practice is well ventilated with a clean flow of air. Avoid dusty or smoky places or places with high amounts of artificial air fresheners. But do not get so fixated on finding a quiet, isolated place; you may not have this as an option and you do not have to wait until this time of space becomes available to practice Pranayama. Make the best of the circumstances and locations that are available to you now.

Precautions and Contraindications

Consult with your physician to make sure that these practices will not negatively affect any underlying conditions. Take a slow step into learning these practices and pay close attention to emotional and physical changes. Do not rush through these exercises. Always promote the habit of breathing through the nostrils unless the exercise requires breathing through the mouth. Avoid any exercise that you cannot physically do. For example, if one nostril is completely blocked from allergies, sinusitis, nasal congestion, etc., you may not be able to practice an exercise involving both the nostrils. Avoid fast breathing exercises during times of active symptoms, for example, asthma. Do not practice Pranayama under the influence of any psychotic substances or alcohol. Generally, use your internal guide (a.k.a. common sense!) to follow your own system and its wellbeing while practicing.

Health Conditions and Medications

Although Pranayama is a systemic practice and can help with symptom management in several diseases, it is not your primary therapeutic tool. It is an adjunct practice that could aid healing. Do not stop your medication without consulting your physician. Not all Pranayama are suitable for every health condition. Every Pranayama is different and the effects can be variable from person to person, and within a person at different times. So be aware of your health conditions, and follow appropriate consultations with a certified Yoga Therapist specialized in Pranayama, along with your physician. Depending upon the practice there might be adjustments required to your prescribed medication, and that will be determined by your physician.

Online Materials and Private Lessons

Some of the Pranayama exercises are available online as videos on my website: Pranascience.com. Please see them under the "Learn" tab. In addition, some of the online courses I conduct will make the videos of the sessions available to the registrants. There are a number of other online sources available for Pranayama although with a limited number of techniques. While referring to those, or for that matter, my own exercises, practice caution as to the authenticity, a reference to the tradition, prior research, experience level of the teacher, plus your own judgment based on several other reference materials. It is always a good idea to take beginning lessons in person from a Pranayama instructor. This will be helpful in terms of an introduction to the right techniques, the theory behind them, learning what to look for when you do a particular exercise, and clarifying any questions you might have. Sometimes private lessons from a certified Yoga Therapist are better if you have specific health conditions that require one-on-one attention. I teach weekly classes, workshops, immersions, and teacher training courses. Check my website for a schedule or contact me if you are interested in learning about or hosting a program near you.

1

Dheerga Swasam (Deep Breathing)

Move the breath

Deep and tall

Move the mind with it

Until you reach a point

They do not move anymore

How To

This exercise is done by breathing in and out through both nostrils simultaneously. Begin by slowly exhaling from the upper chest, then the lower ribs, and then the tummy/abdomen. Once you have completely exhaled to your maximum ability, start slowly breathing in. First, breathe in into the abdominal area. The tummy should bulge out when you breathe in; make sure that the tummy is not tucking inwards. Continue to breathe in moving up, filling up the lower ribs and then the upper chest. Once your chest area is completely filled in, breathe in a bit more all the way up to the collar bone. Once you have inhaled to your maximum capacity, start breathing out from the upper chest, and then move down to relax the lower ribs, and finally the tummy. The key places to watch during both inhalation and exhalation are:

- The upper chest
- The lower ribs
- The tummy

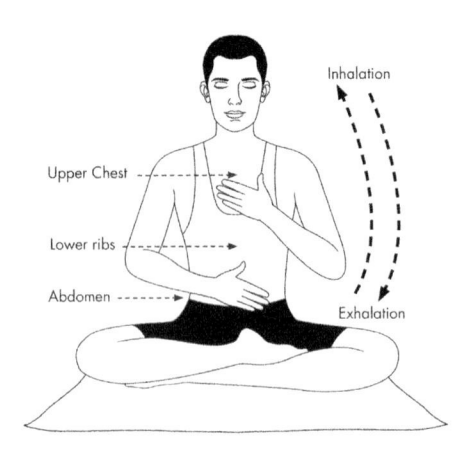

34 | Mind Your Breathing

Dheerga Swasam

We normally take about 12–18 breaths per minute. This changes according to our activity, age, and several other factors. Whatever may be your number at the beginning, try to slow it down as you breathe in and out. The number of breaths can become typically less than seven breaths per minute when you perform this exercise. Make sure you do not focus on the number alone, especially when you start Pranayama for the first time. You have to first get comfortable with watching the breathing and understanding the normal speed of your breathing, and then from there, you try to regulate or slow it down with this exercise.

Another key aspect of this breathing exercise is combining the mind with the breathing. As our mind is a wanderer, it is a challenge to focus on one thing. Breathing is an excellent internal process that can be utilized to bring focus to the mind. Let your mind follow the breathing as you perform this exercise. For instance, you can bring your focus or attention or awareness to the three areas of activity, namely, the upper chest, the lower ribs, and the tummy. Just watch those places sequentially, and continuously as you inhale and exhale. It is normal for your thoughts to move out to something else. But without condemning your mind, bring the focus back to the breathing process and how it moves. With constant practice, you will be able to follow the breathing with your mind.

How Long

You can do this exercise for any length of time as long as you are comfortable with it. If you are breathing fast during this exercise, you may not be able to continue it, and you may want to take a break. It is perfectly all right to take a break whenever you feel it necessary. Your ability to feel physically and mentally comfortable during this exercise is important. Typically anywhere between 5–15 minutes is good for this exercise. In my classes, this is one of the first exercises I teach because this is basic and important for people to understand their own length of the breath, and also the movement of their mind.

Tips

Look for your progression by potentially reducing the number of breaths that you take in a given minute. You will be surprised that you could be taking as low as two breaths a minute. Also, watch how your mind can easily be tamed by watching the breathing.

2
Pranava Pranayama (Om Chanting)

One letter is the beginning and end
It starts and ends with the same sound
It is the background of all the sounds
It connects us all with the One

How To

Begin by breathing in through your nose. Slowly inhale by filling the tummy, then moving upwards to fill the lower ribs and upper chest. Once you are completely filled, open your mouth and start saying the O, as in hOme. As you keep exhaling, continue with the pronunciation of O. And, when you are somewhere in the middle of the exhalation, start closing the lips to make the sound Mmmm…

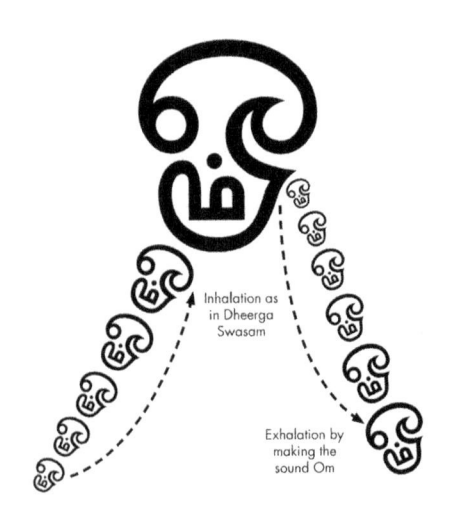

Inhalation as in Dheerga Swasam

Exhalation by making the sound Om

It is a very simple chant; however, there are several details to be aware of. Let us consider a few key points during the chanting of Om.

1. When you begin, never begin with A. Some people chant Om as A… U… M. This is wrong. Aum is part of another chant called Navakkari from Thirumanthiram (It is explained as another exercise within this book. Look for Navakkari chanting. Om chanting has to start with the letter O.

2. When you start with the letter O, the sound should hit the soft palate. Imagine that the sound rises upwards from the throat, hits the roof of your mouth, and vibrates this entire area.

3. The second letter M can be started at three different timings. One, at the very end of the breath. In this way, you will say a very long O all the way up to the end of your breath, and then you will close your lips by saying M for the last few seconds. In the second variation, you will start saying M somewhere in the middle of your exhalation time. This will have a slightly longer M chanting duration than the previous variation. And the third way of chanting OM is by a very short O and then a long M sound.

You can choose any way of chanting the OM. It can vary as you move into the chanting, and it is totally fine if it takes its own form. Once you breathe out completely with the M sound, start breathing in again for the next chant. Make sure that you perform the inhalation through the nose, and exhalation is done by way of chanting. You will notice that during the sound of O, you will breathe out through the mouth, and during the sound of M, you will breathe out through the nose naturally.

How Long

This chanting can be done for any length of time as long as you are comfortable. Generally, keep the chanting for a minimum of three rounds. It can be continued for 5–15 minutes. Sometimes a long O sound and a short M sound will be a good way to stimulate yourself. And, on the other hand, the short O sound, and a long M sound could be a way to calm yourself down. Any method of chanting OM is a good way to regulate the breath, as well as a way to create sound vibrations in the pharyngeal area. I do OM chanting at the beginning and end of most of my classes. I provide an alternative 'Humming' if people are not too comfortable chanting OM as someone might think that it is a religious chant. OM chanting can be done both in the morning and evening or anytime during the day.

Tips and Variations

Think of the soft palate throughout all phases of the chant. You will find that focusing on this area is important in your progression through Pranayama practice, and connecting it with the elevation of your consciousness. This is also a good way to stimulate salivation. Also, controlling the mind is an added benefit of this exercise. Om chanting can be a chant used for Udgeeth Pranayama, which is basically using any chant along with the breathing. This is the basis for my recent audio publication called "Chanting is Pranayama" that you can listen to on several online sources or purchase as a compact disc.

Anuloma Viloma Pranayama (Alternate Nostril Breathing)

Go with the flow
Breathe against the flow
One balances the other
Every side is unique
And, make the life glow longer

How To

Hold your fingers as shown in the diagram/picture. Close one nostril with the thumb. If you use the right hand, the thumb will close your right nostril and vice versa. Breathe in through the other nostril. At the end of inhalation close the left nostril with the little finger and ring finger together and exhale by opening the right. Once the exhalation is complete start breathing into the right nostril to continue the next cycle. Essentially you will be inhaling through one nostril and exhaling through the other. You switch the nostril only when you are at the end of inhalation. Do not switch the fingers at the end of exhalation. Continue the exercise as slow as possible so the breathing is long and deep. As you practice, let the mind travel up and down with the breathing.

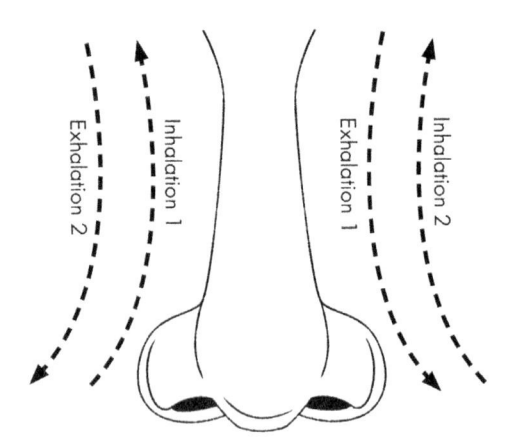

How Long

The ANB (Alternate Nostril Breathing) can be practiced anywhere between 5–25 minutes. As a general rule 10 minutes at any given session will be helpful. This exercise can either be combined with other Pranayama exercises or it can be practiced in isolation. This can be practiced 2–3 times (morning, noon, evening) a day.

Tips for Practice

Keep a constant watch on the nasal cycle. Try to see how you feel during left or right nostril dominant conditions. This may inspire you to do the exercise while watching how the sensations vary. This is because the nasal cycle switches the nostril dominance from one side to the other about every 2–3 hours depending upon the time of the day, and the day of the week. Having a properly alternating nasal cycle is important for good health. The Alternate Nostril Breathing exercise helps to maintain the nasal cycle.

4
Viloma Pranayama (Stepped Alternate Nostril Breathing)

Small steps to the top

Descend in harmony

Reassure that at will

You can control your breath

Because you are the Master

How To

This exercise is very similar to Alternate Nostril Breathing exercise (Exercise #3). However, during this exercise one nostril is used for inhalation and exhalation in a different way. In the word Viloma, the letter "Vi" means opposite. We are going to go against the natural flow of the breath. This is explained below. Read through the complete description before doing it.

In this exercise, there are 2 types of breathing, one for each nostril. The 2 types of breathing are:

1. Long inhalation/exhalation in one smooth action.
2. Inhalation/Exhalation is broken into several parts.

Inhalation

Exhalation

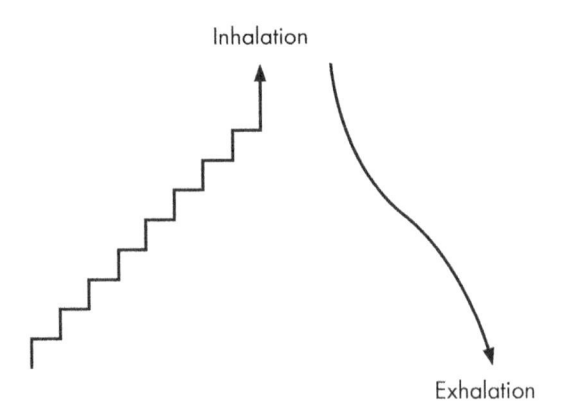

This is explained below for easy understanding. Check which nostril is flowing more freely when compared to the other one. Let us keep this as the "open or active" nostril. The other nostril which has a less open flow is called the "closed or Inactive" nostril. For both inhalation and exhalation through the open/active nostril, perform normal inhalation and exhalation in one smooth action. For example, if you are doing an inhalation through this nostril, inhale as one smooth action, filling up the tummy, the lower ribs, and upper chest areas. Breathing in and out in this nostril will resemble that of Alternate Nostril Breathing.

Regarding the other closed/inactive nostril, both the inhalation and exhalation through this nostril will be a little harder than through the other nostril. Breathing in and out through this nostril is done as small steps. In other words, the one smooth inhalation or exhalation is done in several steps. As you breathe in, perform the inhalation in several small fractions. Imagine how you would go up the stairs. It is one flight of stairs containing numerous steps. Every step is controlled by your ability to control the breathing. You control the inhalation or exhalation in a stepwise manner. Both the inhalation and exhalation through the closed/inactive nostril is done in a stepwise manner.

The sequence of the whole exercise is explained below: (in this example, the right nostril is open/active, and the left nostril is closed/inactive).

1. Close the right nostril with the thumb. Start breathing in through the left nostril as going up the stairs in several steps. Breathe in all the way you could. Actually, at the top of the stairs, you will be able to add a few more steps of inhalation.

2. Close the left nostril, and open the right nostril. Now start breathing out through the right nostril as one smooth exhalation (no steps here). Breathe out completely.

3. Begin inhalation through the right nostril as one smooth continuous flow so you could fill yourself as much as you could.

4. Close the right nostril with the thumb and open the left nostril and start breathing out of the left nostril as going down the stairs in several steps. Breathe out completely by going down the steps and add a few more steps as you descend. All these 4 steps form one full cycle.

5. Go to step 1 to begin the next cycle.

How Long

You could do this exercise at least three times a day (before breakfast, before lunch, and before dinner), each time for about 5–15 minutes. As this exercise is meant to be activating an otherwise dormant nostril it might be better to do this exercise every time the nostril switches (about 2–3 hours interval). However, there is no specific restriction on when to do this exercise.

Tips

As this exercise provides an opportunity to understand the nasal cycle, and also to activate the nostril that is not active at any point, this is a good way to stimulate both the opposing sides of the nasal systems. In addition, breathing muscles-nerves coordination is improved when we practice this exercise. Therefore it will be a good practice to improve the communication between the voluntary ability to control the breath and the muscle groups involved in actual breathing. This exercise could also provide signals to the upper respiratory tract on the nostril dominance, and therefore could activate other signaling to the brain. Keeping these in mind, performing this exercise whenever you would like to achieve control of mind and breath would be beneficial.

Chandra Nadi Pranayama (Left Nostril Breathing)

Calm and quiet

The breath goes on left

Like the full moon

Shining mind is a boon

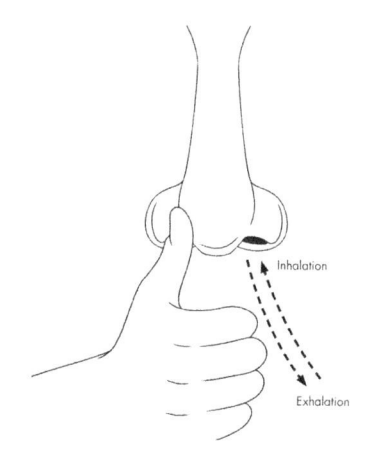

How To

Chandra nadi is also called Ida nadi or the moon nadi that is activated by breathing through the left nostril. It has a cooling effect on the emotional and physical aspects of the system. To activate the Chandra nadi one has to pay attention to certain things. For instance, there may be situations, or conditions in which one could activate it (example, when feeling anxious, being highly agitated, warmed up, hot external temperature, etc.), and in circumstances when you do not want to activate it (when you are already feeling lethargic and unmotivated, as during the time when the temperature is already cold, or during the times of colds/infections).

The way to perform Chandra Nadi Pranayama is quite simple. Close the right nostril (remember, you want to activate the left nostril, so you need to close the right nostril). Start by slowly breathing in, engaging the abdomen, lower ribs and upper chest moving upwards. Once you fill yourself to your maximum ability, start exhaling through the same nostril (left nostril) slowly, by relaxing the upper chest, lower ribs, and the abdomen. Breathe in and out slowly by aligning the mind with the breathing. With every breath in and out, make sure you are able to extend the inhale and exhale to your maximum ability.

How Long

You could do this exercise whenever you would like to relax. You can do this practice until you feel calm. The timing could be as short as 5 minutes. The maximum you can do this exercise is fifteen minutes. Also, it is good to watch the temperature outside and see if you have any cold symptoms. When it is very cold (like in winter) or during times of cold infections, it is better to avoid this Pranayama. Extended periods of the same practice are also not recommended.

Tips and Variations

Do the exercise as slowly as possible, which will provide instantaneous relaxation. Follow the breathing with the mind so that the mindfulness is also improved. Focus your attention into the nasopharyngeal region (or the roof of the mouth or the soft palate) so your mindfulness on every inhalation and exhalation is improved. You could do this exercise either as a single smooth flow for inhalation and exhalation or as stepwise breathing in and out. When you perform the exercise in a stepwise method, both inhalation and exhalation can be divided into several small steps. Always allow your creativity to find alternative ways of practicing, and allow yourself to experience new things that are not mentioned in this book!

6

Surya Nadi Pranayama (Right Nostril Breathing)

Wake up like the morning sun
With zeal and vigour
The mind and body glow
To enlighten the self and others

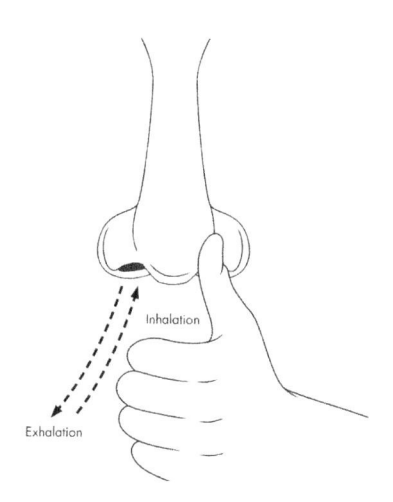

How To

Forced right nostril breathing is how we activate the Surya Nadi. This exercise is to be performed when your right nostril is somewhat blocked for an extended amount of time, or when you want to feel instantaneously energetic and active, or just to get warmed up. That is why the right nostril is called the Surya Nadi or Pingala Nadi.

To do this exercise, close the left nostril using any of the fingers or methods you like. Typically I use the little finger and ring finger on my right hand together to give a complete closure of the left nostril. This allows me to breathe in and out of my right nostril. Now, begin by breathing out, relaxing the upper chest, lower ribs, and the abdomen. Breathe out completely. Then begin by inhaling from bottom to top, by filling the abdomen, lower ribs, and upper chest all the way up to the collar bone. Once you think you are completely full, start exhaling. All the breathing in and out is done through the right nostril. There is no switching of fingers or nostrils in this exercise.

Be aware of the mind and make sure it is following the breathing. Then, become even more aware of the breathing. For instance, you could pay close attention to the following sensations: what is the speed of my breathing; am I breathing fast or slow; how is the temperature of the breath now; am I feeling the breath warmer now; how do I feel emotionally at this time; am I producing more saliva; how do my eyeballs move; is there a stimulation in the scalp or inside of the skull; is there a sensation at the tip of my earlobes, etc. You could ask several questions and follow what happens as you proceed through the practice.

How Long

As this is a warming up exercise, you do not want to force this for a long time. I recommend doing this for five minutes. Based on how you feel, you could take a little break and do it afterward if you need more time. Doing this continuously for longer than 15 minutes is not advisable as this could have a strong effect on the cardiac and emotional systems. The times could very well vary from person to person and within the person, there could be variations depending upon timings. So one has to follow the internal guidance in addition to the general practical guidance provided in this book. If there is any medical condition that concerns you, it is recommended that you consult with your physician to make sure that this exercise will not harm you.

Tips and Variations

I generally do this exercise when I am feeling lethargic or unmotivated, or at times when I feel sleepy in the middle of the day. This could stimulate an awakened and warmed up feeling. You might not have to do Surya Nadi Pranayama when your right nostril is already open and running actively. It is not necessary to blow more into an already open/active channel. Instead, you could do this when the right nostril is not active, or when it has been somewhat blocked for an extended period of time. As mentioned in regards to some of the earlier exercises such as Chandra Nadi Pranayama, you could do this exercise by inhaling and exhaling as steps instead of one straight and smooth inhalation/exhalation. This provides more control of the breathing, mind, and their coordination. Also, when the breathing is pulsatile as in the stepwise breathing, the signals that are provided to the upper respiratory system, especially to the olfactory lobe pathway, could stimulate the brain in a much more profound way. It is like ringing a bell several times instead of just once. Always follow your interoception to determine when to stop, and when you need a little more.

Thirumoolar Pranayama (TMP)

Counting the breaths

The ins, outs, and the stills—

Adds countless days to life

Long and healthy we stay

How To

This exercise is from the ancient Tamil literary work called Thirumanthiram written by Saint Thirumoolar. This is the basis of our most recent research studies showing salivary stimulations with numerous biologically important molecules being activated or regulated with this exercise. If you would like more information, a whole Chapter is dedicated to this exercise in my earlier book "PranaScience: Decoding Yoga Breathing". This exercise involves a timed inhalation, breath-holding, and exhalation. The information on the specific nostrils and timings for each step is the key for the best results.

Thirumoolar Pranayama (TMP) | 51

Inhalation (2 counts)

Nostril opened less

Nostril opened more

Breath-holding (8 counts)

Exhalation (4 counts)

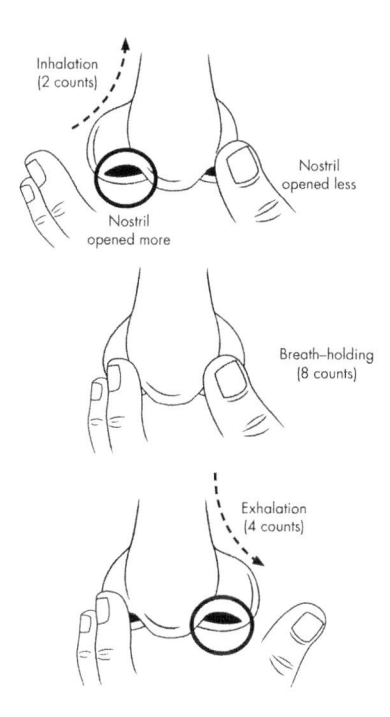

To begin this exercise one has to know which nostril is open/active at this time. You can do this by performing a few rounds of Alternate Nostril Breathing, or by simply breathing in and out of both nostrils. In this example, I am explaining with the assumption that the left nostril is open/active whereas the right nostril is a bit closed/inactive. So the inhalation is through the left nostril, then there is a breath-holding, and the exhalation is going to be through the right nostril. Each step is timed, and the time is kept not by numbers but rather by chanting length. For example, if you say 'Om Namasivaya,' the length is about eight mathirai, based on Tamil literature. You could use any chant you would like, something around this length (for example 'I'm relaxed,' 'I'm beautiful,' 'I'm peaceful,' etc. are some other examples). Chant this within your mind twice to time the inhalation length. This should allow you to fill yourself completely. At the end of inhalation, close both nostrils and hold the breath for eight counts of the same chant within your mind. This might be challenging at the beginning, but one can build up the capacity to hold the breath for this long. Once the breath-hold is complete, open the right nostril (in this example), and exhale for a length of four counts of the chant. This should help with complete exhalation. Once you exhaled completely, begin inhaling from the left nostril to start the next cycle. Essentially the cycle goes in a circular fashion (not alternating through the nostrils), meaning the inhalation and exhalation in this exercise are always through the specific nostrils (left or right).

How Long

The exercise is best performed for a minimum of 10 minutes. The suggested timing for this exercise is 24 minutes (one nazhigai) by Saint Thirumoolar. Three times per day (once in the morning, once in the middle of the day, and once in the evening) would be good times to do the exercise. The factors that we stimulate in the saliva could appear in as little as five minutes. But certain factors might take longer to show up. Therefore it is good to do the exercise for longer than five minutes and up to 24 minutes. Also, the factors that are produced could be reduced to normal/basal levels after some time. So it is important to re-stimulate the system by performing the exercises again.

Tips

If you do not exhale fully, you cannot inhale fully. Therefore focus on the exhalation so it is complete. Then you will be able to inhale fully. Once the inhalation is full, then you will be able to hold it for a good amount of time. This exercise is useful when you are experiencing uncontrollable sneezing due to sudden allergic exposure. Also, this is a good one to stimulate salivation and several factors thereof. Please refer to my research papers on my website PranaScience.com.

8
Kukriya Pranayama (Panting Breathing)

Drive away those impurities
Cleanse again and repeat
Just by the breath
No more blemishes

How To

This is a funny looking exercise. The first and foremost thing that you need to get yourself ready for is that you should not have any inhibition to do this exercise. This involves opening the mouth widely, stretching the tongue out, and breathing. Altogether it may make you look quite silly.

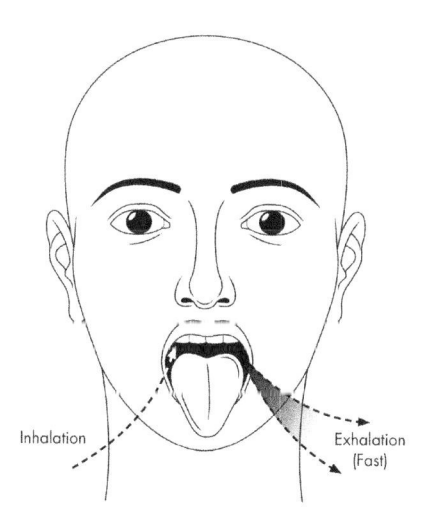

Inhalation   Exhalation (Fast)

You can do this exercise while seated or while standing up and bending forward with both hands on both knees for support. Begin by opening the mouth and stretching the tongue out. Then start breathing out through the mouth. At this time generate the exhalation from the tummy area. Extend the exhalation as much as you can. It does not have to be a sharp exhalation, rather it could be a complete exhalation starting with a burst and then following like a trail all the way until you complete the full exhalation. Once you have exhaled to the maximum, breathe in through the mouth with a natural pace. You do not have to emphasize on the inhalation. Only the exhalation is powerful. Let the inhalation proceed at a normal speed as it flows. Once the inhalation is complete, exhale forcefully as before. You can do this exercise for about 10–30 cycles. Always start with a low number and work your way up. Each round will consist of about 10–30 cycles of inhalation/exhalation. After one round, take a few normal breaths to allow yourself some time to rest. And then continue with another round. You can do a total of 3 rounds with sufficient rest in between.

How Long

The whole process of doing three rounds of 30 cycles in each round might take up to 5–10 minutes depending upon the resting periods in between. The exercise can be done once in the morning and once in the evening for three rounds in each sitting. Fewer numbers of cycles, with a reduced number of rounds, can also be helpful. For example, two rounds, each with 10 cycles with three normal breathing in between rounds could be helpful in quickly experiencing a cleansed feeling. The breathing exercises, most of the time, do not have an upper limit for practice time as long as they can be done with ease and comfort.

Tips

With every exhalation, you could imagine that something that you do not want in your physical or emotional system is going away. This could provide a sense of cleansing to your mind and body. This can also stimulate the soft palate area and can have an instant effect on the central nervous system. I like to do this exercise when I feel that I have accumulated a lot of impurities in my body, especially through breathing, for example after going through a dusty area. I have also done this in situations when I have felt to have impurities in my mind or thoughts. This exercise is a reassuring one to cleanse us and to reset us to the previous clean mode.

Kapalabhati (Shining Skull)

Like a fire the breath raises
Brighter gets the soul
With the light of breath
The veils of the mind burn

How To

This is also called Shining Skull as it is supposed to have a prominent effect on the skull/brain. You may want to have some tissue handy during this exercise as it involves an action similar to blowing the nose (funny one again!). Every exhalation is forceful through the nostrils. Followed by every exhalation, there is inhalation, but the inhalation is slow, normal and not very active. Begin the exercise by focusing on the tip of the nostril or the lower part of the abdomen. Start breathing out in one big spurt through the nostril. The force for breathing out starts at the lower abdomen. Tuck the tummy in, to generate the necessary power to force the air out. As the air moves out you could focus on the tip of the nostril. It is perfectly fine to keep the awareness in any location you would like. However, the emphasis is on the diaphragm muscle contraction to push the air out, which is achieved by pulling the tummy inwards. While every exhalation is forceful, every inhalation is done in a relaxed fashion, basically allowing the inhalation to proceed without much effort. Relaxing the tummy after the forced exhalation will allow the inhalation to proceed almost automatically. One exhalation followed by one inhalation constitutes one cycle. One could do anywhere between 30–60 cycles at a stretch to finish one round.

At the end of a round, take a nice deep inhalation through the nostrils at the desired pace as required, and hold it for as long as you can. At the end of the breath-hold, breathe out and watch the breathing. At this time you could choose a particular place within your body (say the middle of the forehead or top of the scalp) to send your breathing to and from as you watch the breathing. This is a brief relaxation period.

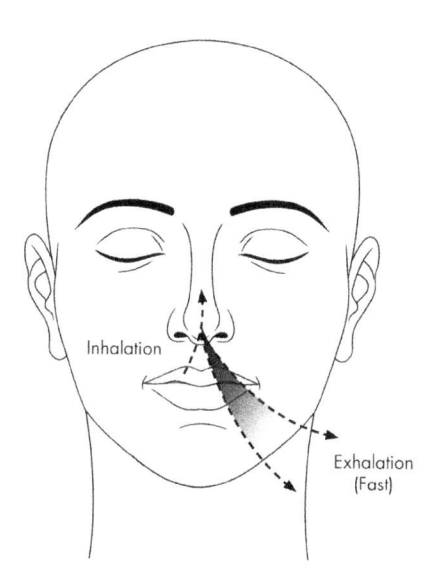

Inhalation

Exhalation (Fast)

After the relaxation step, perform another round of 30–60 cycles as mentioned before. At the end of the cycles, perform the breath-holding as mentioned before. You could do a total of three rounds with sufficient time to relax in between.

How Long

Kapalabhati can be done for three cycles twice a day (once in the morning and once in the evening). The cycles can be shorter, and the number of total rounds can be fewer, too. If you exhale or inhale too vigorously some lightheadedness may occur. Be watchful about any lightheadedness and stop the exercise when any discomfort is felt. Continue with normal breathing. You could continue the exercise at a later time or the next day.

Tips and Variations

Kapalabhati can be done with very mild to medium to strong exhalations. This can be done as mild as normal breathing. Make sure that the tummy is not full. It is not ideal to do this exercise after a heavy meal. Also, having a lot of undigested food might produce a similar discomfort like lightheadedness. So it is better to look for our own responses to the exercise by initially performing a few rounds. Always we need to remember that the body changes continuously, and therefore it is important to look for our responses to any exercise by frequently testing the exercise on it at possible variations.

Bhastrika (Bellows of Breath)

Chase the horse of breath

As fast as you can

After a sprint you will see

How easy it is to meditate

How To

This is one of the fast breathing exercises, and can potentially cause lightheadedness. Caution must be exercised to know your limits and not overdo it. It is recommended that one should start with a few cycles and a few rounds and then build up as you move further. In addition, the ideal days and times for Pranayama practice may vary; the same exercise in terms of length and strength might be acceptable one day but not the next. So it is important to understand the current state of your body and mind and to test a few cycles before one enters into longer practice. Also, those with some active symptoms (for example those with breathing troubles like asthma) should make sure that there is no current shortness of breath while doing this exercise.

In this exercise both the breathing in and out are active. We forcefully exhale and then immediately inhale with the same vigour and speed. The length of inhalation and exhalation are almost the same. Sometimes it can be long or short depending upon how fast we do this exercise (see under for Tips and Variations).

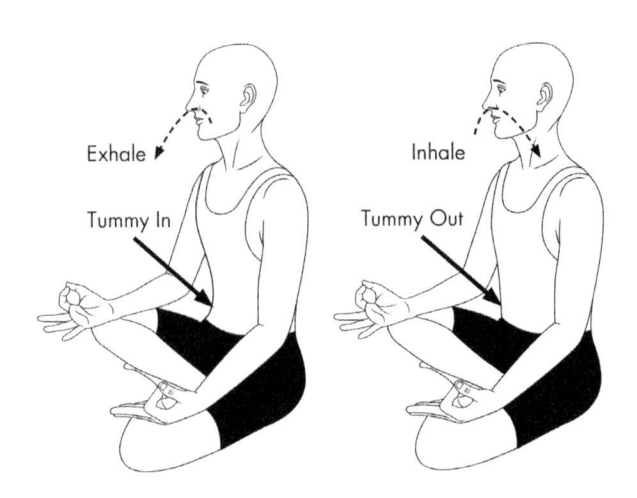

Begin by exhaling forcefully from the top of the chest all the way to the abdomen. Tuck the tummy in as you breathe out completely. Then swiftly breathe in filling upwards, from the abdomen to the top of the chest. As this is a fast exercise, you will not be spending much time filling the lower ribs. The transition at that point is very quick. That is the reason I mention only the two parts – the upper chest and the abdomen. Inhale all the way up to the collarbone as quickly as you can, and then start the next exhalation. There is some sense of rapidity in this exercise. There is no pause between the inhalation and exhalation. Do this for 10–60 cycles as per your comfort level. That is one round. At the end of the round take a deep breath and hold the breath as long as you can. At the end of this breath-hold, release and watch the breathing. Take enough rest to feel the effect of the exercise and to get ready for the next round. You can do up to three rounds at a given time.

How Long

The three rounds of Bhastrika can be done twice a day (once in the morning and once in the evening). A mid-day session could be included depending upon the exertion level. If someone is physically exhausted, or exposed to extremely hot weather, then it might be better to avoid a mid-day session. The three rounds could contain any number of cycles from 10–60 depending upon the comfort level of the practitioner. This exercise has a calming effect on the respiratory stimulation so you won't be breathing in and out heavily immediately following the exercise. Because of this reason, Bhastrika is one of the exercises performed just before meditation as a way to calm the breathing which will be helpful in meditation.

Tips and Variations

If you get any lightheadedness from this exercise, try it another time or another day for a few more attempts. Normally doing this on an empty stomach might be helpful to reduce any lightheadedness related issues, or generally for all the Pranayama practices. The key variations are short breaths versus long breaths in every cycle. The breathing can be as short as possible; which will allow you to breathe several times during one round. If you are doing extended inhalations and exhalations the number of breaths within a round could be less. Both long and short variations are good to practice. Initially, it might be better to start with the long variation and then progress to the shorter version.

Variations related to movements of the hands: During this exercise, there is active involvement of the muscles involved in breathing, including the muscles of the shoulders. Movement of the shoulders and the arms will help aid the breathing process. Stretching the arms sideways as you breathe in, and bringing them forward as you breathe out is one way of coordinating the breathing with the movement of the arms. The other way is to raise one hand straight above the head while the other one is folded at the sides of the hip/chest. This is for the inhalation step. And, for exhalation the hands are switched, the folded hand goes up, and the uplifted hand is folded to the side of the chest. You could bring more variations into these shoulder/arm movements. The synchrony is important to maintain during the inhalation and exhalation.

Agnisara Kriya (Fire Rising)

The fire rises from the root
It churns and burns the impurities
And lightens up the nadis
Gives a day that is bright and clear

How To

This exercise can stimulate the Mooladhara (root chakra) along with the other two base chakras, namely, the Swadhittanam and Manipurakam. These three lower chakras are key in generating a sense of warmth. Therefore engaging them in this exercise is supposed to be a good way to stimulate a warm feeling both physically and mentally.

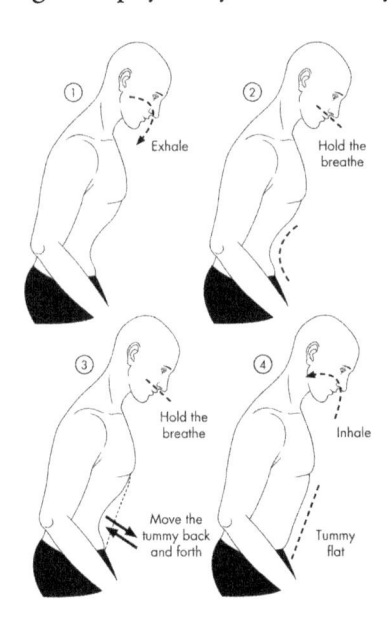

This exercise is normally done by standing up with a slight forward bend; the hands rest on both the knees to give support. The breathing is through the nostrils. Begin by breathing out starting by relaxing the upper chest, the lower ribs and then the abdomen. Once you reach the abdomen for exhalation, increase the force of exhalation and empty out all the air you can. At the end of exhalation hold the breath out; meaning that you are not going to inhale immediately. Rather move the belly in and out (tucking and releasing actions) several times. Remember during this movement, there is no inhalation or exhalation; the breath is being held. Once you are done with the movement of the belly, start breathing in through the nostrils and stand upright to watch the breathing. You can close your eyes. Or you could use the mountain pose (Tadasana). That was one round. You could do up to three rounds for a complete exercise. The number of inhalation/exhalation cycles one completes depends upon one's own ability. So please follow your internal sensations to extend the exercise to suit your timings.

Tips and Variations

One could do these exercises by sitting in a sukhasana or any comfortable seated pose as long as the breathing through the belly is uninterrupted. There is a possibility that the exercise will stimulate the bandhas (techniques involving locks at the chakras). While it is not necessary to activate the bandhas, it might not be a concern if the bandhas occur spontaneously. However, there should be enough attention to the abdomen and then the whole system.

12

Sudharsana Chakra Kriya (Solar Plexus Exercise)

Inhale and hold
From the gut
Raises the hidden power
To fill you with determination

How To

I learned this exercise from one of the courses I attended with Anmol Mehta. I owe this exercise to him and the tradition of Kundalini Yoga practice. I encourage everyone to check out his online classes and web resources on his website (AnmolMehta.com). Please remember that the general rule for almost all Pranayama exercises is that the stomach should be empty before starting the exercise. That is one of the reasons that the Pranayama is suggested to be practiced in the early mornings. Also, this is one of the exercises that require a proper seated pose, no lying down or walking!

Sudharsana Chakra Kriya (Solar Plexus Exercise) | 65

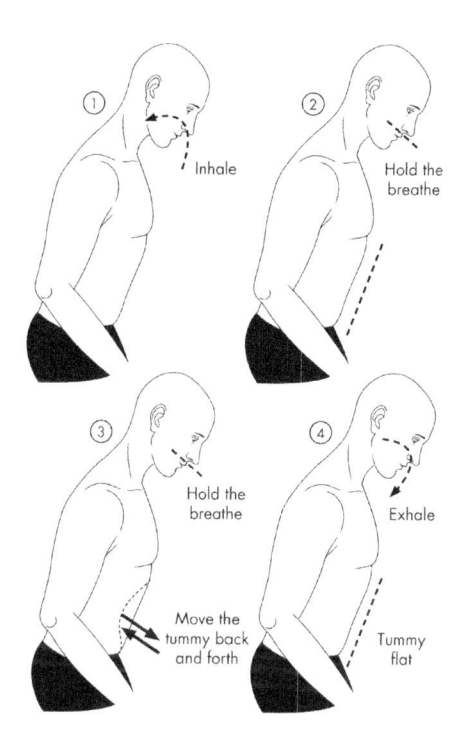

To begin the exercise, breathe out completely through the nostrils. Then close the right nostril and breathe in through the left nostril to fill yourself all the way. At the end of inhalation, hold the breath until all of the following actions are completed: pull the tummy inwards, imagine the navel approaches the spine, in one strong action; release the tummy; repeat this for 8, or multiples of 8 (16, 24, etc.); every time you pull in the tummy chant a mantra of your choice within your mind (that is right, you cannot chant loud when you are holding the breath!). The Kundalini Yoga practice suggests Wahe Guru (praising the Guru). The point of using a chant is to focus the mind and body on the pulling action and for synchronicity. I use the chant Om Namasivaya repeated four times in a tune so I can do the counting easily. Once all the eight or multiples, pulling actions are completed, close the left nostril and breathe out of the right nostril. This is one cycle of the exercise. Perform this for 3–11 times. At the end of each cycle, one could take a brief rest if desired.

How Long

Doing this exercise 3–11 times is a good starting point. This should take about 5–15 minutes for the whole exercise depending upon your resting time in between. Performing the exercise once in the morning and once in the evening is suffice. Making sure that the tummy is free of any undigested food is key to feeling good at the end of the exercise.

Tips and Variations

One key variation to this practice is the number of pulling actions we do per each mantra chanting. Each pulling action in the above example is just one strong motion of the navel towards the spine. In the variations, this action could be divided into two or three smaller motions for each mantra chanting. In other words, during each mantra chant going on in your mind, pull the tummy inwards half a distance first and the remaining half the next if you are doing two pulling actions. If you are doing three pulling actions within one chant then you pull the tummy thrice during the single chant, each pulling action would approximately cover a third of the total extent; and you would do three such pulls for the complete inward motion of the navel towards the spine. Holding the breath for a longer time during this practice could be challenging when you go high in the number of pulling actions, or in the multiples of three, or in the combination of the two. The best way is to go easy and gradually build the numbers up. Do not overdo it to a level that you feel pressure building above your neck. Always know your comfort zone and stay within.

Thee Moochu (Breath of Fire)

Short bursts of breath
Flutter like a butterfly
Fly around warm and active
Wake up the fire within

How To

This again is an important exercise in the practice of Kundalini Yoga. This is used along with several kriya practices (involving the powerful movement of breath, muscles, postures, rituals and chants). Generally, the practice of a Yoga posture with normal awareness of breathing can be replaced by the breath of fire breathing. This exercise, due to its vigorous nature, is considered one of the fast breathing exercises, and it is said to stimulate the Mooladhara chakra to raise the power within the Kundalini. Explaining Kundalini is beyond the scope of this book.

The breath of fire exercise as the name says is one way to sense the heat that can be produced just by altering the breathing. This involves rapid inhalation and exhalation through the nostrils. This might look like the practice of Bhastrika that is explained in Chapter 10. However, it is different from Bhastrika in that the length of each individual inhalation and exhalation in the breath of fire exercise is very short making this exercise more rapid than Bhastrika. As this exercise can be combined with several physical and mental forms and actions, there is no specific posture necessary to practice. For the purpose of learning, it can be practiced with the seated cross-legged pose.

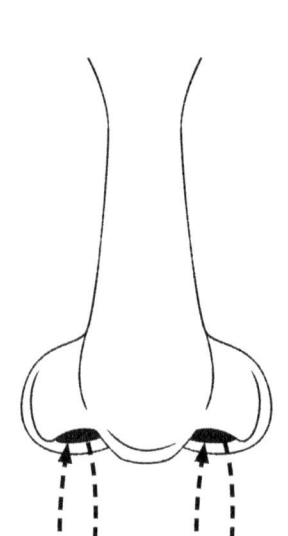

Short bursts of inhalation and exhalation done fast

To begin the exercise, start by breathing out halfway so that at least half of the air remains inside. At this point start breathing in and out rapidly in short spurts of inhalation and exhalation. Focus your breath on the tip of the nostrils. Depending upon the time for which one could keep doing this action, the inhalation/exhalation cycle comes to a halt somewhere within one minute. Once the cycle is complete come to normal breathing and watch the breathing. All the inhalations and exhalations are around the same length.

How Long

Repeat this cycle for 3–11 times with intermittent breaks to watch the breathing. It might take up to 5–15 minutes for the exercise. This can be done not just in the morning and evening, but also during the day whenever there is a need for us to get activated or warmed up. This gives instantaneous activation to break any lethargic cycle.

Tips and Variations

Initially getting a rhythm of equal inhalation and exhalation could be challenging. Also, every breath can appear longer than we want. However, one can master this technique after several weeks of practice. As mentioned earlier, breath of fire can be combined with several postures and rituals. After learning the technique thoroughly to get the inhalation and exhalation equally, you could incorporate it carefully into your other practices. Attention to specific posture and space for doing the breath of fire practice is important.

14
Ujjayi (Ocean Sound Breathing)

The secrets of the heaven

Poured into you in a hissing voice

Way to the fountain of joy and peace

And the key to new doors

How To

Ujjayi is a well-known exercise among numerous Yoga schools. However, the power or the ultimate goal of Ujjayi is not as widely understood. In the Siddha philosophy, the soft palate (also called Annakku in Tamil) is an important anatomical location. This is considered the path to the Sahasrathalam (crown). This place is best activated by the breath and the mind together. Either one alone would be unable to activate the same response. Because this area is considered as something that will "open up" the Sahasrathalam to enable communication with the Vignanamaya kottam, or with the skies, it is considered very important. Sahasrathalam is called Uchi in Tamil and in the Siddha philosophy. because of its ability to open up, this exercise, the Uchi is called the Uchi Pranayama. This could have become what is now called Ujjayi Pranayama.

Ujjayi (Ocean Sound Breathing) | 71

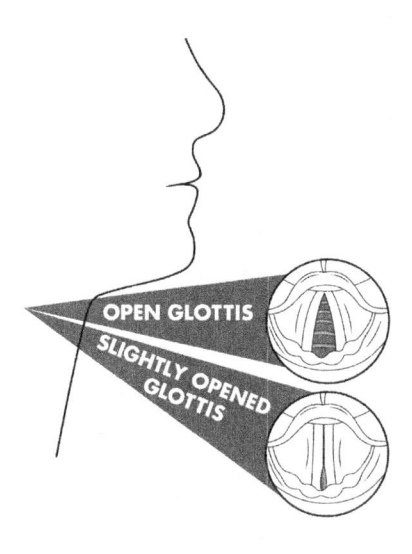

OPEN GLOTTIS

SLIGHTLY OPENED GLOTTIS

This exercise is done by allowing the air to pass through the vocal cords with some constriction applied by the movement of the laryngeal muscles. Consider saying the word "ha" by opening the mouth; it will be similar to a hissing sound. By the middle of the sound, continue the sound but with the mouth closed. Now the sound comes from the throat as always, but the air escapes through the nostrils. This is how the Ujjayi sound is generated. The sound resembles the ocean or the noise you hear when you hold a large seashell up to your ear. Once you are able to produce the sound, continue with a comfortably long inhalation and exhalation. It is not absolutely necessary to equate the inhalation and exhalation. Let them flow freely. The main idea here is to listen to the sound of the ocean and keep the inhalations and exhalations as long as possible.

The key though is to look into the Annakku (the soft palate), and breath in and out through this region. After several breaths, it will bring a slow realization of the crown chakra (Uchi). You might feel several of the following: a sensation at the middle of the forehead, stimulation of the nerves all around the scalp radially; stimulation of nerves at the top of the scalp; and coordination of breath and the pulse above the middle of the forehead.

Tips and Variations

This is a wonderful practice to do before and during meditation. It is easy to start a meditation class with Ujjayi breathing as this is something that can quickly bring the focus to breathing, and then to meditation. Watching the middle of the forehead and top of the head are important.

There are a few variations of the practice depending upon the position of the tongue. In one variation we could keep the tongue relaxed and resting on the oral floor. The other option is to raise the tongue so it touches the soft palate, near Annakku. This gives a burning sensation after some time. Some people might want to release the tongue after a few minutes because it might be painful to keep the tongue stretched. Whatever works for you is good. Touching the soft palate with the tip of the tongue is a way of indicating a place where the mind and breath can be watched together. This will help us solidify our meditative practice.

15

Bhramari (Humming Bee Breathing)

Goddess of black bees

In the forest of time

Hums and flies

To Her tunes we dance.

How To

Bhramari in Hindu mythology is the Goddess of black bees. The humming of the bee sounds like a chant, Reem. The word Reem is a specialized chant as part of Navakkari chanting. The Tamil word Reengaram refers to the sound of the bee. This exercise is nothing but humming like a bee with a bit of breathing regulation. The humming bee sound that connects us with the Brahmam can also be called the Bhramari. This exercise involves deep breathing and humming accompanied by a mudra.

SHANMUKHI MUDRA

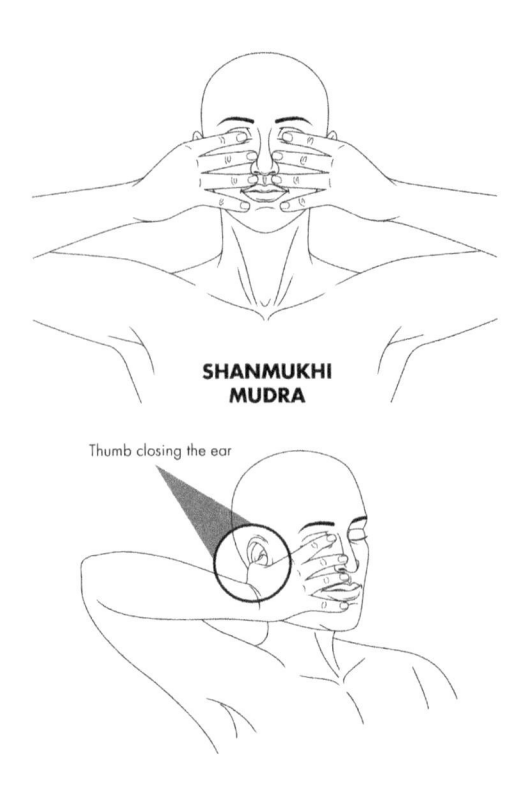

Thumb closing the ear

For this practice, the fingers in both hands are organized in the following manner. You may want to plug the ears with earplugs and to close the eyes. If using the hands for the mudra, the fingers are arranged in the following manner. Please note that the fingers are just set on those places without putting too much pressure: the hands are put together with the fingers touching the respective fingers on the other hand, except the thumb and index fingers. The little fingers in both hands touch each other, and so on. The thumbs are kept apart. Both the little fingers are set below the lower lips, the ring fingers above the upper lips, the middle finger above the nostrils, the index fingers are set apart and kept on each eye, and finally, the thumbs are used to plug each ear. It is perfectly fine to do it without the fingers in this posture.

After the fingers are in this position, take a deep breath through the nostrils, and exhale as a humming. The humming will create a reverberating sound inside the skull with a nice vibration depending upon the tone. Listen to the sound of the humming made possible through the closure of the ears. Breathe out as much as you can by humming out. After the complete exhalation/humming, begin by breathing in using the method of Dheerga Swasam (Chapter 1), i.e., by inhaling as slowly as possible engaging the tummy, lower ribs and upper chest filling from the bottom to the top. At the end of the inhalation, begin humming to start the next cycle. Continue this cycle listening to the humming sounds. The hands stay in the mudra throughout the exercise.

How Long

The Brahmari breathing can be done for any length of time as long as you are feeling comfortable. Normally any time between 5–10 minutes would be an ideal duration for this exercise.

Tips and Variations

The tone of the humming can be anywhere between the deep down (for example, C in C major scale) to an upper pitch (for example, B in C major scale). The choice could be depending upon the vibration area one would like to feel inside the head. The lower pitches would produce vibrations at places different from those produced by the upper pitches. Also, the lower pitches and upper pitches would vary in frequency of vibration as well. There are some interesting variations one could apply to the humming. That includes the following: instead of pronouncing the letters m during exhalation, one could pronounce the letters Nnnnn or Llllll, or Iiiii, or Rrrr..., Vvvvv, Ng..., Nj..., Zh..., etc. during exhalations. This creates a different set of vibrations in the tongue, upper palate, and in the head. These are variations that I have discovered during my practice. The exact mechanisms by which these could influence the physical and mental state are not yet clear. However, the variations could be as powerful as Brahmari.

16
Savithri Pranayama (Rectangular Breathing)

Measure and carve
Beautiful like a box
Confine the breath
Master the art of control

How To

Having a good control on the breathing apparatus, namely the ribs, the intercostal muscles, and the diaphragm is important for maintaining the breathing capacity as we age or as the breathing machinery wears out. Also, the control of mind over the breathing process helps one to maintain good voluntary control on the breathing while also helping with emotional regulation. Savithri Pranayama is a breath-holding exercise that has multiple advantages including that it provides an opportunity to 1. Watch the breathing as a meditation, 2. Control the breathing, 3. Hold the breath both inside and outside, 4. complete all of these processes without the involvement of hands, and 5. Develop control of the breathing process.

```
                    Holding (breath held in)

            ↑                              ↓
            |                              |
            |    Inhalation    Exhalation  |
            |                              |
            |                              ↓

                    Holding (breath held out)
```

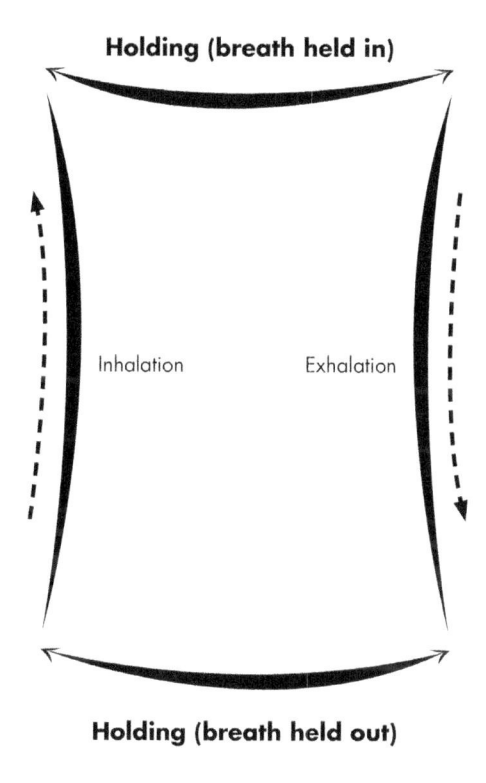

To do the exercise one has to get familiarized with some way of counting so we can follow the length of inhalation, exhalation, holding in, and holding out. My favorite way of counting is chanting a repetitive mantra with a tune within my mind. I use a pack of four "Om Namasivaya" as a tune. When I say these four chants, it lasts approximately 4–6 seconds. Chanting it with the same pace will keep the counting almost the same throughout the practice.

The lengths for the breath-holding phases are half the length of both inhalation and exhalation. So, we will have two lengths, one full length (for example eight counts of the chants), and the other one is half-length (four counts of the chant). 1) At the beginning of the exercise, we breathe out for eight counts. 2) At the end of exhalation, wait for four counts (holding the breath out). 3) At the end of the four counts, breathe in slowly beginning to fill up the abdomen, and moving upwards for eight counts. 4) At the end of full inhalation that is typically spread throughout the eight counts, hold the breath for four counts (holding the breath in). After this breath-hold, go back to step 1 to start exhalation for a period of eight counts.

How Long

This can be done for a period of any length as long as one is comfortable. Normally 5–15 minutes is a good length to observe an effect. This exercise can be done any time during the day irrespective of where you are. The key is that there should be enough space in the abdomen to accommodate a complete inhalation, exhalation, and holding.

Tips

Savithri Pranayama is a good practice for the workplace, especially in jobs that require extended sitting, and for places where other people are around or if you are concerned with using your hands or postures to do the exercise. It might be difficult to do the exercise, especially when holding the breath out. There would be a rush to breathe in after the breath-holding out. This is an important place to practice the mind control of breathing. Taking a break after any of the four steps would make it easier to learn the exercise. It is better to start with low numbers, say for example 6-3-6-3, and then slowly build up to higher counts. Practice will make it perfect.

Sama Vritti (Balanced Breathing)

Balancing the breath
The mind gets balanced
When everything is balanced
No ups and no downs

How To

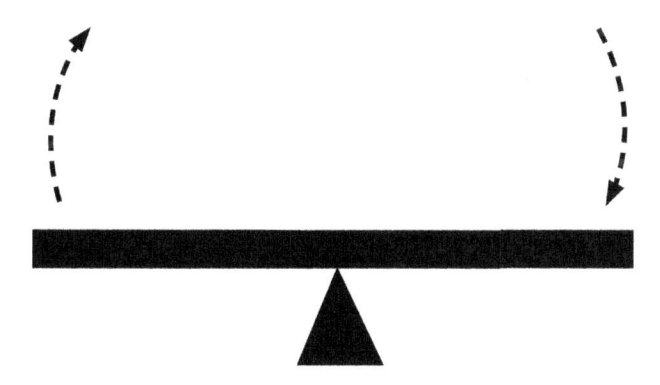

Balanced inhalation and exhalation

This is Equal Breathing or balanced breathing. It is simple, yet very powerful in gaining control over the breathing. This could also bring a good balance to the physical and mental components because the inhalation/exhalation equality might bring a good acid/base balance in the blood.

Begin by exhaling for a specific length of time or number of counts. Once the exhalation is complete, without any major pause or breath-holding, begin inhaling for the same duration of time by engaging in counting/chanting.

Continue this for several minutes or for as long as you are comfortable; watching the breathing intermittently at your own pace, taking a break when necessary.

Tips

Use chanting numbers or tunes to equate the breathing in and out. That would make this a good meditative experience. Slowly extend the numbers by increasing both the exhalations and inhalations equally. Even a mild single number inhalation and exhalation would be a good practice to slowly improve the breathing.

18
Vishama Vritti (1:2 Breathing)

Take in less
Give out more
Makes you healthy
Wealthy, and wise

How To

This is one of the breathing methods that could bring instantaneous relaxation and control over the mind. As the name says, it involves exhalation two times longer than the inhalation. While normal breathing involves a slightly longer exhalation, this exercise emphasizes an extended exhalation.

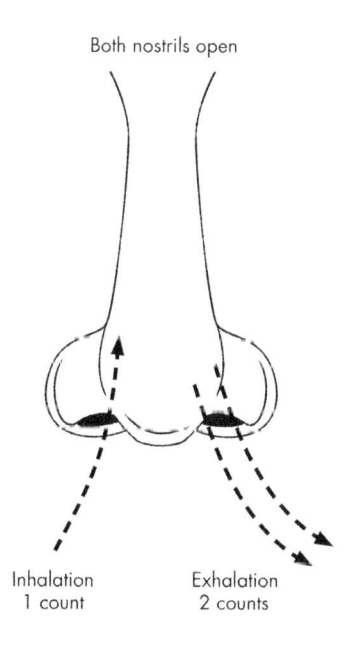

Both nostrils open

Inhalation
1 count

Exhalation
2 counts

To begin the exercise, exhale completely, without any counts, and then start the inhalation with a specific count, let's say four chants. Next, start exhaling for eight chants. You could pick any numbers that you are comfortable with for the inhalation and exhalation steps.

How Long

Although breathing in and out at different lengths of time for a longer duration of time can create some imbalances in the acid-base in the body, it is also a way to activate the kidneys to compensate for these changes. However, performing this exercise for 5–15 minutes at a given time is a good range.

Tips

Do this exercise when you would like to relax and focus on yourself. After a few rounds of this exercise, one could feel calmer. Do not overexert yourself by having longer counts than your comfort level.

Nan Madi Moochu (Four Part Breathing)

Ascend and descend
Four steps each way
Expands the breath wider
And, builds a stronger you

How To

This is one of the exercises to maintain the functions of the respiratory muscles, the neuronal communications, voluntary control over breathing, mindfulness of breathing, and to maintain the overall lung function and capacity.

In this exercise both the inhalation and exhalation are divided into four parts. The complete inhalation goes in four quarters instead of one single inhalation. And the same is true for the exhalation. During inhalation, there is an equal thrust given to each part. However, the fourth inhalation could take a little longer to fill completely. In the same way, the exhalation is divided into equal parts whereas the last exhalation is a bit longer in order to do a complete/maximum exhalation.

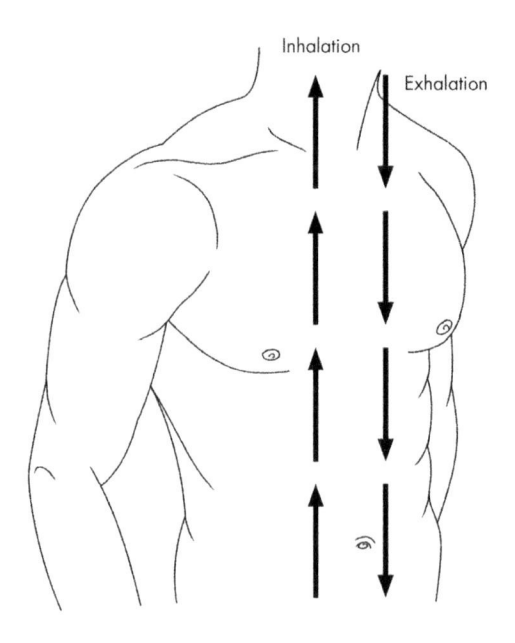

To begin the practice, start by exhaling in four parts. At the end of complete exhalation, begin inhalation split into four parts. There is no pause between inhalation and exhalation. Since this could be a fast way of breathing, there is a chance of hyperventilation. So it is important to keep watching the comfort level and to remain aware of any lightheadedness if it arises.

Tips and Variations

It might be a good idea to associate the accessory muscles during this exercise. For instance, stretch both the arms forward, and then start swinging them sideways in four stepwise movements coordinating with four parts of inhalation. And, bring the arms to the front in four steps coordinating with four parts of exhalations. This will coordinate the breathing with the muscular movement. The other option is to hold the hands together in front of the chest pushing one palm over the other. This generates some stability to the breathing process during the exercise.

20
Padi Moochu (Multistep Breathing)

Up or down
One step at a time
Makes a long journey feasible
With grace and control

How To

This is essentially the same type of exercise as the Alternate Nostril Breathing. However, the movement of both inhalation and exhalation follows a pattern similar to going up or down a staircase. For the breathing exercise, we should be able to close and open the nostrils alternatively using the fingers similar to the technique used during the Alternate Nostril Breathing exercise.

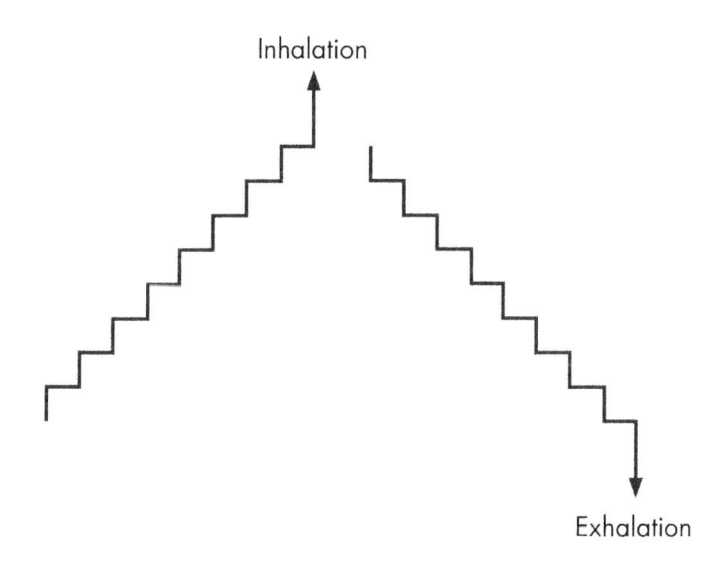

Inhalation

Exhalation

Begin by closing the right nostril and breathe out through the left nostril slowly in a stepwise manner. Imagine the exhalation happening in several steps instead of one smooth exhalation. You can adjust the number of steps according to your comfort level. Typically about 10–20 steps can be a normal range. At the end of exhalation, inhale through the left nostril in the same stepwise fashion. Each inhalation and exhalation have the possibility of extending beyond the normal ability. Once the inhalation through the left nostril is complete, switch the nostrils by closing the left nostril and opening the right nostril and begin to breathe out in a stepwise manner. Essentially, this is inhaling and exhaling in a stepwise fashion by alternating the nostrils.

In this exercise, the emphasis is given to the steps in each inhalation and exhalation; and also to the extent of deeper inhalation and more complete exhalation. This allows for control over the breathing and therefore the mind.

How Long

This exercise can be done for 5–15 minutes for several cycles as long as one is feeling comfortable. Watch for any physical or mental changes. You can do this both in the morning and evening or during the day time whenever there is a need for controlling the breath.

Tips

Every inhalation or exhalation can be coupled with a short mantra, for example, Muruha, Om Shanthi, Siva, or anything that you would like that is short enough to match it to the stepwise breathing, several times during the inhalation and several times during the exhalation.

Pongu Moochu (Fountain Breathing)

The Ganga is within you
Know the fountainhead
Make the paths clear
The elixir begins to flow

How To

This exercise requires a bit of imagination and it has a profound effect on one's mindfulness in breathing. Also, it has a great impact on elevating consciousness through breathing.

This exercise can be done by keeping the eyes closed or opened. The breathing is through both nostrils and there is no involvement of fingers unless you would like to use a mudra during the exercise. Begin by breathing in through the nostrils as slowly as possible. There is absolutely no need for very deep breathing like the Dheerga Swasam. However, as you breathe in, imagine that the inhalation is completely engaging the abdomen, lower ribs, and the upper chest. The timing for total inhalation is the time for the breath to start somewhere in the root chakra (Mooladharam) and move upwards to reach the crown chakra (Sahasrathalam). You can also imagine that the inhalation arises from the Mooladharam and passes through Swathittanam, Manipurakam, Anahatham, Visuthi, and Agna chakras. Once the inhalation is full, begin the exhalation through the nostrils while imagining that the breath is going out through the crown chakra just like a fountain. Slowly breathe out to the maximum possible extent as slowly as possible. Once the exhalation is complete, move your awareness to the root chakra and begin the next round of inhalation. To summarize this exercise, the inhalation starts at the root chakra and moves up filling the entire chest and abdomen, and finally reaches the crown chakra. Once at the crown chakra, breathe out through the crown chakra. You will have a complete awareness of the breath and the crown chakra, the scalp and the complete circle around the scalp. You may be able to feel the sensation around the scalp. After several rounds of breathing, you can feel that the breathing gets a bit shallower, which is normal.

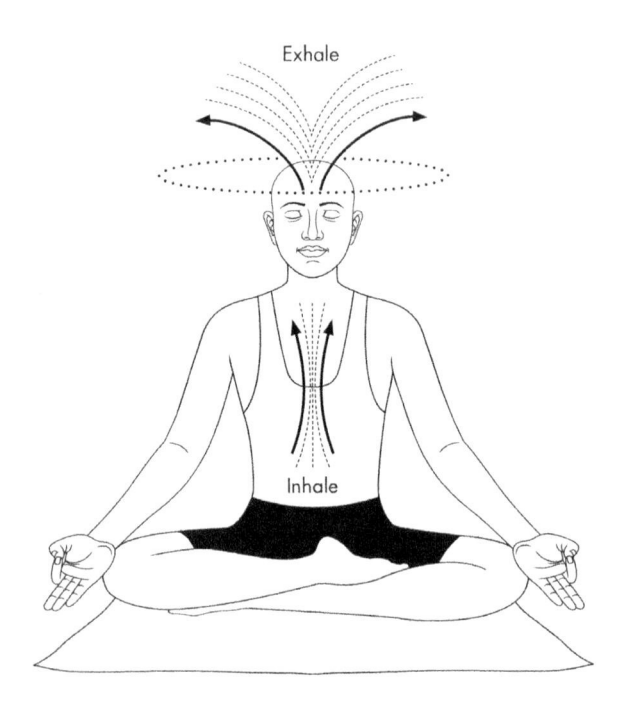

How Long

This exercise is a meditative one and it cannot be assigned a particular time for practice. However, as the breathing involved in this exercise is deep breathing, it might be good to monitor how one feels and change the timings of practice to suit one's needs. It would take at least five minutes to reach the complete sensation of the "fountain" I am talking about. It may take a shorter or longer amount of time for some; that is totally fine. However, once you get to a comfortable zone of inhaling the breath upwards with awareness, and then exhaling out of the crown chakra, you can sustain the practice as long as you are comfortable with it. The breathing rate can be adjusted according to your comfort level. This might slow down further and the breathing might get shallower as you get into a meditative state with this exercise. Allow yourself to return to natural breathing once you reach this stage and enjoy the ride!

22

Ahavoli Moochu (Illuminating Heart Breathing)

Fill the heart with Prana
The heart overflows with love
Joy, and peace
The light illuminates all in the path

How To

I owe this exercise to two wonderful teachers and traditions. The first one is one of my Gurus Nischala Joy Devi that has kindly given the Foreword to this book. I attended her "Yoga of the Heart and Cancer" course, a 10-day course at the beautiful Shri Swami Satchidananda Ashram, Yogaville, Virginia. During that course, I had the opportunity to learn the importance of meditating from the heart in addition to the traditional practice of Agna chakra. The importance she gives to the heart chakra was very well appreciated by every attendee. That gave me an opportunity to combine Pranayama with the heart chakra which I incorporated into my subsequent practice and teaching. The second one is the organization called Sahaj Marg that practices Heartfulness meditation. The name Heartfulness rather than the usual mantra of Mindfulness resonates with me. I got an introduction to Uma K'Sri, an instructor from Columbia, SC. Uma and I spoke over the phone and he explained the practice and we started practicing together over the phone. It is such a fantastic experience to meditate upon the heart. As someone obsessed with Pranayama I discover a way to add a breathing component to any of the exercises or activities. So I explored the possibility of using various breathing patterns into my own Heartfulness practice.

I have found that using breathwork to approach the heart seems to work beautifully. With that little introduction let me share with you one of the exercises I found fascinating to reach the center of the heart through Pranayama.

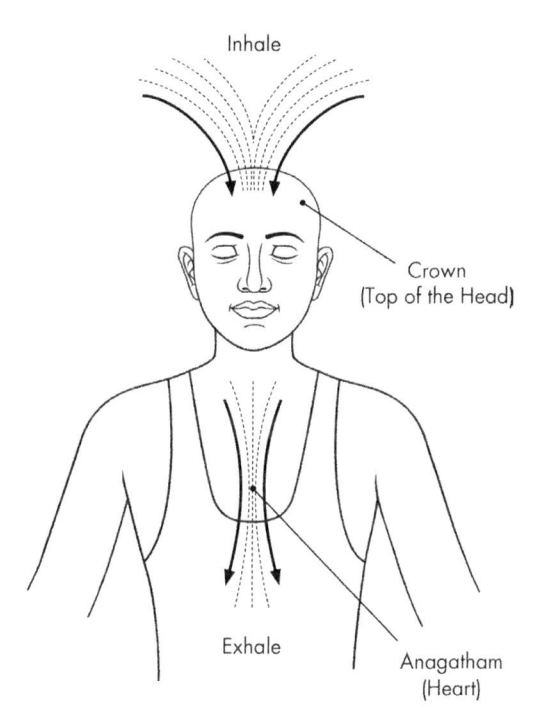

Inhale

Crown (Top of the Head)

Exhale

Anagatham (Heart)

The breathing pattern for this exercise is something like a funnel. Imagine that the bottom tip of the funnel is at the position of the heart, whereas the top collecting portion of the funnel is at the crown chakra or the rim around the scalp. The idea is that the crown chakra along with the rim of the scalp together, like a funnel, collects the energy/Prana from the space as we breathe in, and then pours it into the heart as we exhale into the heart center. The heart will be filled with the energy, broadness, light, and compassion that it collects from the sky above. And, of course, this practice requires the use of the imagination!

This exercise can be done in any posture or while engaged in any activity. However, during the learning phases of this exercise, it might be a good idea to do it in a sitting posture with closed eyes so it will be easy to imagine and comprehend the exercise and all the actions. Begin the exercise with a slow deep inhalation. At the beginning and all the way till the end of the inhalation, let your awareness be on the crown chakra, top of the head, and the rim around the scalp. Imagine that the whole area is receiving the breath or the Prana energy from the sky above. Inhale slowly and smoothly as much as you can. It is ok if the awareness drifts between the torso and the crown during this step, but the ultimate goal is to keep the complete awareness on the crown chakra. Once the inhalation is complete, begin a slow exhalation as your awareness slowly descends passing through the Agna chakra (forehead), and the Visuthi chakra (neck) to reach the Anahatha chakra (heart) where the complete exhalation is poured out. Imagine that you are pouring all the energy you gathered at the crown chakra into the heart during the exhalation. Extend the exhalation as long as you can and enjoy the warm feeling at the heart center, and also notice the feeling of being filled at the heart. With longer exhalations into the heart center, you can experience the overflowing of energy, love, and warmth. At the end of exhalation, begin the next round of inhalation from the crown chakra.

How Long

This can be done as a meditation, so there are no specific timings as long as one is comfortable with the exercise. The breathing can be shortened to a normal pace as one goes into the practice. Whenever your heart needs more energy, love, light, or anything else to fill it up, the Prana can take the form of this need and fill the heart space. In this way, Prana is multitudinous, shapeless, infinite, and can take the shape of anything—energy, love, light, joy, peace, truth, and so on. It is like the box that the Little Prince got from the pilot *(Here is the box, the type of goat you want is inside this box)*. Prana is like that —it can be the medium or content of anything you want to receive from the sky above. With every inhalation the object you wish for flows in, and with every exhalation, it fills and overflows your heart.

Tips and Variations

Do this whenever you would like a positive boost to the heart. There are so many ways you can incorporate breathing into the heart center. Some of the variations are given below: 1) Breathing in and out of the heart, just centering all the breathing within the heart center is another variation. 2) Another could be, not only personally receiving the energy from the sky, but also sending that energy to others. You can achieve this by imagining that you are radiating the breath out of the heart. Inhalation can be from above through the crown chakra, and the exhalation goes out of the heart chakra into the space near you, to your neighbors, to anyone around you, to the globe, to the infinity of the universe.

Pidari Marga Moochu (Back Route Breathing)

The trained horse of Prana
Takes the back routes
To the top of the mountain
To be one with the skies

This is yet another way of practicing Pranayama for improving breath awareness and also for elevating consciousness. The movement of the breath is imagined or sensed as if the inhalation originates in the Mooladharam (root chakra) and then moves upward through the spine (not necessarily the frontal route that engages the diaphragm, lower ribs, and upper chest). And then is finally exhaled through the Agna chakra (middle of the forehead) and the Crown chakra (sahasrathalam).

In the learning phase of the practice, it is better to choose a seated posture with closed eyes. After getting a good grasp on the technique this can be done on the go and even with the eyes opened.

Exhale through Agna and Crown

Inhale through the spine

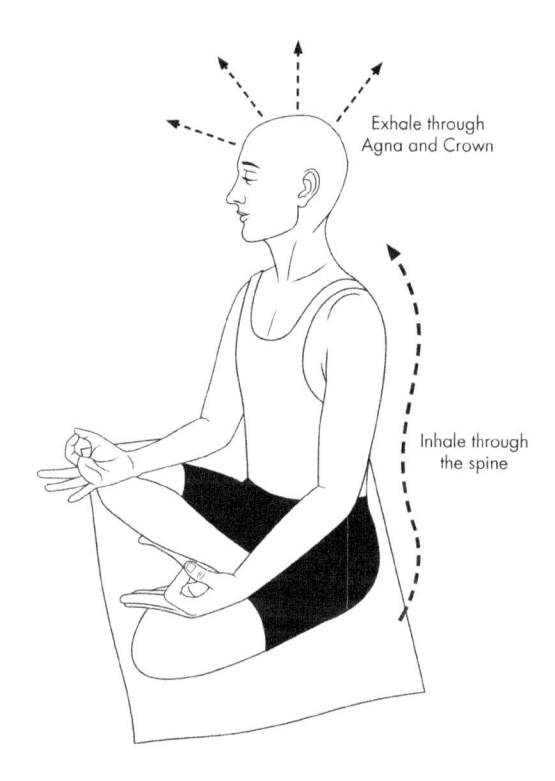

To begin the exercise, exhale completely, and begin inhaling starting from the Mooladharam. Complete awareness at the very beginning of the inhalation has to be at this root chakra, and then as the inhalation progresses it moves up the spine. Once the breath awareness reaches the top of the back, it has to move up through the back of the neck (not through the front), and the exhalation begins at the back of the head and extends all the way up into the Agna and Crown chakras. The exhalation is extended as much as possible until a silent pause in breathing is attained. At this stage, begin the next inhalation from the Mooladhara chakra and continue the next cycle of exercise.

How Long

As with all the other meditative breathing exercises, it is up to the practitioner to determine the length of time for this exercise. The key is the awareness of inhalation, the back route at the neck and the exhalation through the top chakras. Breathing might get shallower or softer as one moves into a meditative stage.

Tips

One thing that might improve the awareness of this exercise is to think of the back of the body throughout the inhalation. While most of the breathing exercises are focused on the diaphragm, chest, all the way up to the nostrils, this is the only one that focuses on the back (dorsal) side of our body, all the way from Mooladhara chakra to the top of the head.

24

Puyal Moochu (Storm Breathing)

It can be silent

Or at times violent

Train it at your will

All are plays of nature

This is a fun exercise that I came up with one rainy morning when I was listening to the sound of the wind blowing outside. I tried to mimic the sound of the wind. It started like Ujjayi breathing, and then as I moved my lips to create different sounds (mainly A and U sounds), I found these minor adjustments altered the flow of the air within the oral cavity, and more especially to the pharyngeal region, and at the soft palate. This let me explore more into the sounds of A and U within Om chanting. That is, you could start an Om chant, and in the middle, you could switch to A and U sounds. I think people chanting Om as Aum may not be correct because Aum is a different chant as I repeatedly say. The possibility of the existence of A and U within Om can be experienced by including A and U in the middle of the chant, not beginning with A. The benefit of doing this exercise could be to improve the feedback of breathing to the brain, to notice how slow and relaxing it is, so the brain can work on tasks stress-free.

Inhale through the nostrils

Exhale through the mouth

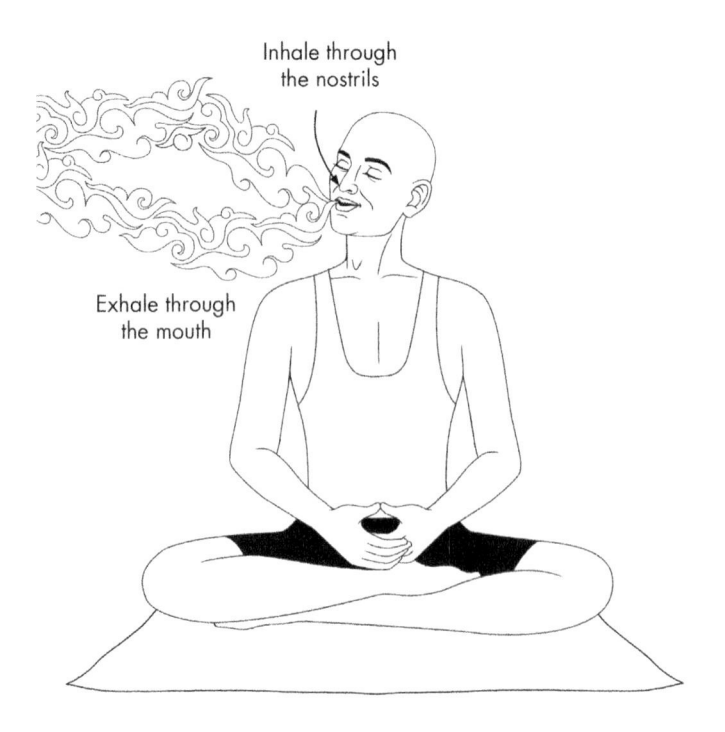

How To

Begin with a deep inhalation through the nostrils. You could do this just like the deep breathing (Dheerga Swasam) engaging the abdomen, lower ribs, and chest. At the end of the inhalation, open the mouth to exhale slowly with the awareness to create a sound similar to a storm. This would be something like Ujjayi or the ocean sound breathing. If you pronounce the word Haaaa that is how it would sound. Once you have started producing this sound, then you can move your lips together to bring a sound Uuuu. Sustain this sound as long as you would like, there is no specific time duration. When you want to switch to the Aaaa sound simply bring the lips sideways as if you are smiling, that will create the Aaaa sound. Be creative! You could make more variations of the sounds. Be aware of the deep inhalation and enjoy the complete awareness during the exhalation at the top of the palate. Once you finish the exhalation, close the mouth and begin the next inhalation through the nostrils.

How Long

Actually, the length of this exercise is not studied in detail. But considering the flow of air through the mouth, and its opened position during breathing, it might be better to do this exercise for any duration less than 5 minutes (any longer may cause dryness in the mouth). Also, the physiological effects of prolonged exhalation into the soft palate region with large volumes of air, as in this exercise, is not well understood. So practice caution to look for any immediate changes in the mood or body conditions.

25
Mandhira Moochu (Mantra Breathing)

Mantras, your personal guide
Like a walking stick,
Leads your breath
In slow steps to proficiency

Mindfulness can be easily cultivated by watching the breathing. In addition to merely watching the breathing, if one could incorporate a mantra or any short phrase, that will add more value to the practice. When repetitive prayers are incorporated into meditative practices, the mind can be tamed quicker, and the inward journey becomes easier. This exercise is about incorporating mantras into the breathing.

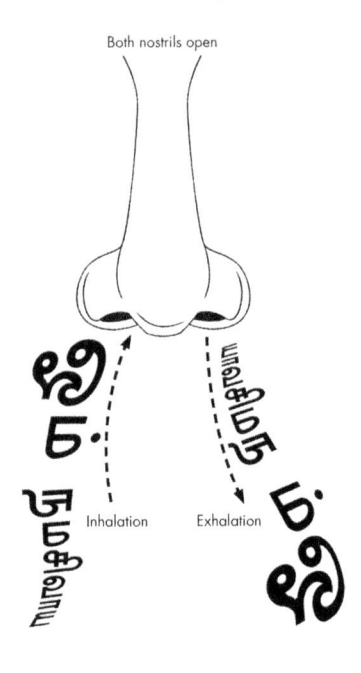

How To

To begin the exercise, choose a favorite chant. For instance, Om Namasivaya is one of my favorite mantras. This can be chanted slow or fast depending upon how you would like to incorporate this into the breathing. Sometimes you might want to repeat the chant slowly so it lasts for the whole breath, or just the inhalation or exhalation, and at other times you can repeat the chant several times within one breath or during the inhalation or exhalation. You will see in the following example how the Om Namasivaya chant is used once during inhalation, and once during exhalation.

Start with an exhalation. Breathe out all the air you can by tucking the tummy in. At the end of exhalation, begin the inhalation from the Mooladhara chakra, and simultaneously begin chanting within your mind as slowly as you can. Move the breathing upwards by filling the abdomen, lower ribs, and then the upper chest. As you move up with the inhalation, you will be chanting in the following order:

Om – Mooladharam

Na – Lower part of the abdomen

Ma – Navel

Si – Lower ribs

Va – Heart

Ya – Up to the neck

Once the inhalation is complete, then begin the exhalation by chanting the same Mantra. Now the letters may not correspond to exactly the same position as indicated above, but instead, they will be in the reverse order as follows:

Om – Up to the neck

Na – Heart

Ma – Lower ribs

Si – Navel

Va – Lower part of the abdomen

Ya – Mooladharam

The last letter during both inhalation and exhalation can be extended to match the length of the breath. Once the exhalation is complete, begin the next round of inhalation as mentioned above.

How Long

This exercise makes the normal Dheerga Swasam exercise into a more meditative one. The timing can be 5–15 minutes, and the breathing pace can be altered as per the demand. This can be done any time during the day at least 2 hours after your last meal; this will allow you to breathe easier than you would if your stomach were full.

Tips

There are several variations including the chant, the length of each chant, how many times one chants during the inhalation or exhalation, etc. Some of the variations are given below:

1. Chant only for inhalation and watch the quietness of the breath during the exhalation. You can do this in the reverse order, i.e., chanting during exhalation and watching the inhalation quietly.

2. Have a tune for the chant. If you could include a tune to accompany the chanting along with the breathing exercise that will add another dimension to the practice, and the length of the inhalation or exhalation can be altered based on the preference of the practitioner.

3. Let the music come from outside too. In addition to listening to an internal chant, one could listen to chanting music, and try to incorporate the breathing on to it. For instance, the Thirukkural album that we produced in our Tamil Sangam would be a fitting tune to listen to. Or even musical works without any words could be another choice where one could listen to the movement of the breath and the music together. Well, when I try to close my eyes and practice this in my kids' school music recitals I get elbowed by my wife that thinks I am sleeping!

26
Sheetali Pranayama (Rolling Tongue Breathing)

Flow of cold breeze
Soothes and relaxes
Stimulates and nourishes
Way to rejuvenate

This is one of the widely popular Pranayama among several schools. This is known as the cooling breath for its relaxation effects. However, upon careful examination of the exercise with respect to the muscular movements, the dynamics of air, and the presence of cells along the way for mechanical signaling, I have included several details into this exercise in my classes.

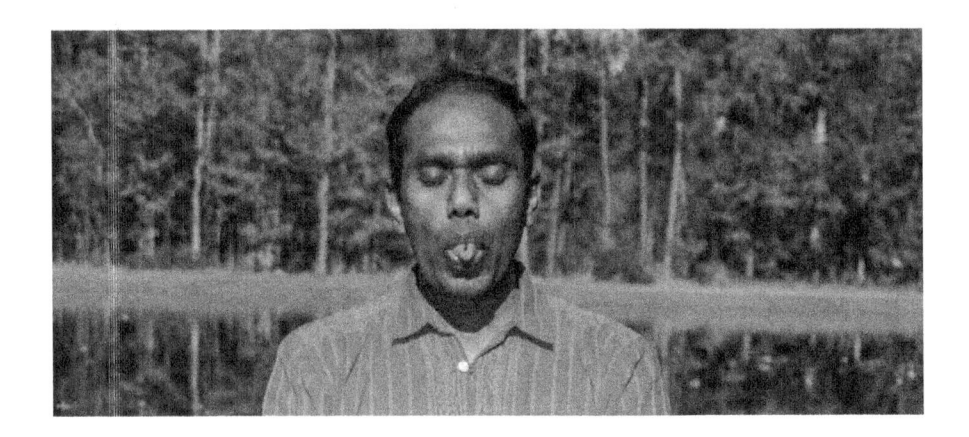

Some of the key points are:

1. The air that goes through the rolled tongue will impinge on the pharyngeal region. This is the place of importance in consciousness and also for the stimulation of various activities in the brain that could potentially be activated due to the targeting of air into this area. In fact, this could be a potential route for stimulating crown chakra neurons, and also salivation. This could also be one of the ways to stimulate secretions from the sinuses.

2. The rolling of the tongue produces torsional/mechanical stimuli on to the tongue muscles, and that stimulation might induce salivation.

3. The flow of air on the surface of the tongue could activate mechanical signaling due to the shear stress on tongue cells, thus stimulating their secretion. This could be very well true for the air induced stimulation of palatine tonsils (normally called tonsils) that could produce more immune response boosting molecules.

As found in my research, salivary stimulation contains several factors that would impact our health. Thus, there is a combination of several beneficial actions within this breathing exercise.

How To

This exercise requires rolling the tongue into a shape almost like a tube as shown in the picture. Some people might not be able to roll the tongue like this. In those cases one could use a straw set on the tongue or the lips can be brought in like the form of O so the air can be targeted on to the tongue. Begin by inhaling through the mouth through the rolled tongue, and fill up to the upper chest. Once the inhalation is complete, pull the tongue in and close the mouth, and then exhale slowly through the nostrils. The exhalation starts from the upper chest and then moves downwards to the lower ribs and the abdomen. Once the exhalation is complete, start the next cycle by inhaling through the rolled tongue.

How Long

This exercise can create a cooling effect on both the physical and emotional states. It might be better to avoid this exercise during extreme cold climatic conditions and during common cold or allergy related symptoms. This will create a sense of cooling and relaxation within about 5 minutes of doing this exercise. Longer durations can be done with caution for any lightheadedness. Also, it may not be necessary to do this exercise for longer than 10 minutes.

Tips and Variations

During the exercise, pay close attention to the tip of the tongue, all the spots in the oral cavity that air goes through, and the lower temperature of the air sensed in those parts. This will improve the mindfulness of the breathing exercise. Also, bringing awareness to the salivation might be helpful to increase the salivary secretion as well. There is one variation to the exercise where instead of rolling the tongue longitudinally on a long axis like a tube, one could fold it so the tip of the tongue folds back to the top of the tongue. At this point, one can breathe in and out as mentioned above for the exercise. The sensations can be felt in different locations compared to the classical Sheetali practice.

27

Sheetkari Pranayama (Smiling Breathing)

In joy we smile, that
Takes away the pain
Brings new friends
Adds more beauty

This is one of the fun exercises that I always do when teaching children because this exercise will make you look like you are smiling during the inhalation. Similar to the Sheetali Pranayama exercise described in the previous Chapter, the inhalation during this exercise has a wide range of spots where the inhaled air due to the shear stress and force can activate salivary stimulation in over 400 minor salivary glands located all over the oral cavity including the gums and tongue. Previous research has shown that these glands can produce numerous bioactive substances that could potentially work on several pathways including pain, immune response and stress reduction. Particularly I would like to point out the connection I found with the action during this exercise, and the action we make in response to an anticipated pain, for example, a flu shot. During the needle stick, we open the lips as if smiling, close our eyes, and inhale through the mouth (or at least we did this as kids). This could be one way of stimulating some stress relieving molecules in response to the pain. Or they could even be pain reducing molecules that we produce.

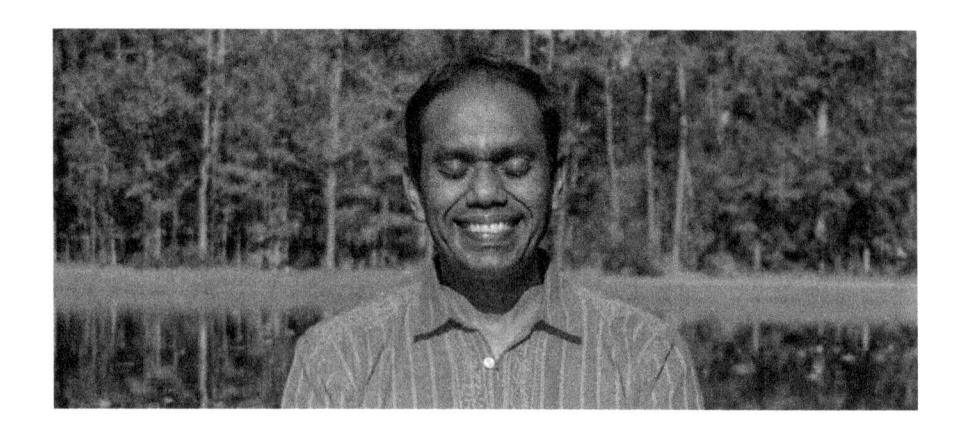

How To

Exhale completely through the nostrils and tuck the tummy in. Begin inhaling through the mouth starting from the Mooladhara chakra and moving upwards; and, simultaneously open the lips wide to show the teeth similar to a smiling action. The inhalation goes in through the mouth, the teeth, and the gaps between the upper and lower jaws. The air first gets squeezed as it moves through the inter-teeth space, and then it expands into the center of the oral cavity. This creates a cooling sensation on the tongue and in the middle of the oral cavity including the palates. Pay close attention to the places where the air touches. Also, take notice of the drop in the temperature and speed of the air. Once the inhalation is complete, close the mouth and begin the exhalation through the nostrils. Perform a complete exhalation starting from the upper chest, moving downwards all the way to the tucking of the abdomen inward. At the end of the exhalation, begin the next inhalation through the mouth while smiling!

How Long

All the rules that apply to the Sheetali Pranayama could be true here including the symptoms of cold, and low-temperature climatic conditions. Also, one might feel sensitivity to the teeth if there are any dental implants or sensitive areas. So care must be taken not to stimulate excessive pain. In some cases, the exercise could cause dry mouth and dry lips as there is a rapid movement of air during this exercise. Again, these responses should be followed along with other physical and emotional status changes and should be taken into account to determine the length of the practice.

Tips and Variations

It is a good idea to think some happy thoughts as you smile and inhale! Under certain conditions, the action of smiling may be difficult to perform. This could be a physical condition or a situation related to your surroundings. In those cases, any small opening that is possible through the slightly opened lips could be sufficient to feel the cooling sensation and to produce relaxation and salivation.

28

Sithan Pokku Moochu (Sithar's Way Breathing)

அறிவொன்றற நின்றறிவார் அறிவில்
பிறிவொன்றற நின்ற பிரானலையோ

He stands persistently in the wisdom of those
That have the realization
Beyond the boundaries of knowledge

— **Arunagirinathar**

The practice of Pranayama offers numerous ways in which we can regulate our breathing, and each breathing exercise has some benefits. We have seen in this book that various exercises have the ability to impact the respiratory system and some exercises help us promote watching the mind. Pranayama can also be a tool to regulate our level of consciousness. We have the ability to move our consciousness beyond our body, our mere breathing, the mind, and even beyond our wisdom. This transcendence of our consciousness is towards a state of blissfulness. This is the stage where, as Arunagirinathar in the above two lines says, that the Lord is there constantly in the wisdom of those who stay in a state that their consciousness has dropped or crossed the boundaries of the wisdom sheath. While numerous texts talk about elevating consciousness, transcendence, and blissful states, there has been no clear technical guide that I have come across other than ancient Siddhar poems that lays out this path. Especially Siddhars like Kakapujandar, Karuvurar, Pambaati, and Kuthambai have indicated the technique in subtle ways that one can put together. It is like making a dish from bits and pieces of recipes from different books. I was able to put together the present form of this exercise to the best of my understanding solely due to the grace of my Gurus, and that is the reason I name it Sithan Pokku (the way of Sithar). This also denotes that this is not the final form of the exercise; rather it is a continuously evolving one and will be a key to open several doors depending upon our practice and will-power.

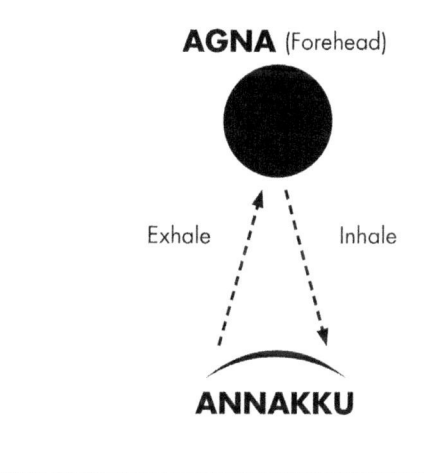

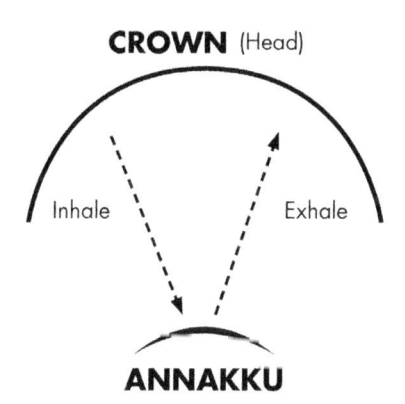

AGNA (Forehead)

Exhale   Inhale

ANNAKKU

CROWN (Head)

Inhale   Exhale

ANNAKKU

How To

Technique-wise there are a few important things we need to be aware of here; which have mostly been covered in the earlier exercises in this book.

For this exercise one needs to have a cultivated awareness to 1) breathing, 2) location of Annakku (the soft palate, the naso/oropharyngeal region, 3) Agna chakra (middle of the forehead), 4) Sahasrathalam (crown chakra), and most importantly, 5) the possible sensation of an Annakku connecting Agna and Sahasrathalam. In this process of awareness, imagination can initially provide us with a rough sketch, on to which further roads are built with practice.

In the initial stages of practice, it is better to try the exercise with the eyes closed. As you become more advanced in your practice, you can try it with eyes opened. Practicing with closed eyes brings awareness to the Annakku. I always refer to Annakku as the combination of naso and oropharyngeal regions. If you would like to bring instant awareness to this spot, just fold your tongue and touch the top of the soft palate. This is the topmost part of the roof of the mouth. That is the region you are going to focus on during this exercise. You do not have to keep the tongue up, you can release the tongue whenever you gain the sensation of the location of the Annakku. With the awareness on Annakku, sense the breathing in that area. You can forget the nostrils, the chest or abdomen during this breathing. Once you are aware of the breathing, gently allow the breath to exhale through the Agna. Of course, your breathing goes in and out of the nostrils, but you imagine that the exhalation goes out of the Agna. After a few breaths, begin imagining that the inhalation comes in from the Agna, too. So the Agna is going to be the source of inhalation and the destination of exhalation. Now you have successfully connected your breath with the Agna. Practice this for several days or weeks. Once you are comfortable with the Agna, then move your awareness to the crown chakra and make that as your new destination for exhalation, and source of inhalation. I could have made the Agna and Sahasrathala routes into two different exercises, I put them as one to show the evolving nature of this exercise. This can elevate one's consciousness, and it depends upon the practice.

How Long

This can be a state where you can be for as long as you would like. While there is no upper limit for how long this can be done, and anecdotes say that sages have gone into meditation for years without food or water, we need to be careful on choosing the target goal for the practice—am I looking for Samadhi, or am I merely practicing to lead my present life more happy and healthy. Setting an alarm, for say 30 minutes to 2 hours could be a good choice. And I would suggest that 30 minutes to 2 hours is the desired range of practice time for today's lifestyle and to take care of chores at home! This can be done every day in the morning or evening.

Tips and Variations

Once you have a good handle of the awareness of the breath in those areas mentioned above in the exercise, you could begin practicing in places like the bus stop, airport, or grocery store lines with normal looking eyes. This practice also has a few stages. In the first stage, you will practice by looking at a non-moving object. The eyes may be looking at the object, but they are completely turned inwards. There is no information going into your mind about the object that you are seeing, but rather you are making an internal journey with your breathing. The next stage is even more fun – your eyes do not have to remain static on one object. They can move to look around and to be aware of the surroundings, but your internal breath and awareness are on the Annakku-Agna-Sahasrathala route. And, you will be surprised that you can find more forms of your own existence beyond what we call the body and mind.

29
Vizhi Nokku Moochu (Gaze-Controlled Breathing)

The breath listens to your gaze
Like a lover it reads your eyes
With no words it follows your orders
Goes left right up and down

In this practice, one will be able to use the awareness along with the movement of the eyeballs for performing the Alternate Nostril Breathing exercise. At the level of breathing, it might not be the same as the traditional Alternate Nostril Breathing exercise, but with regard to cultivating the awareness of the nasal cycle, this is an important exercise.

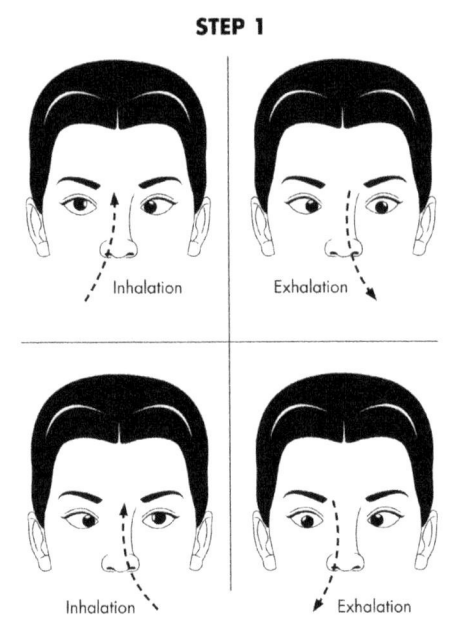

STEP 1

Inhalation   Exhalation

Inhalation   Exhalation

STEP 2

How To

Close your eyes. Keep the palms in the Gnana mudra or cling the fingers together on the lap all throughout the exercise. Begin by mentally scanning the nostrils at the level of the tip of each nostril. Then begin inhaling through the nostrils slowly and with complete attention on the nostrils. Gaze through the closed eyes to the tip of the left nostril. As the inhalation goes deeper raise the gaze along the left nostril all the way into the left eye. This would be at the top of the inhalation. At this stage when you are ready to exhale, switch the gaze to the right eye, and then begin breathing out through the right nostril. Remember, only the gaze through the closed eyes and the awareness are on the right nostril. The hands are not involved in the switching of the nostrils. Obviously, there will be air passing through the nostrils during both inhalation and exhalation. However, it is the awareness that makes the exercise special and sets it apart from the traditional Alternate Nostril Breathing exercise. At the end of exhalation through the right nostril, begin inhalation through the right nostril, moving towards the right eye along the right nostril so as to reach the right eye at the end of inhalation. Once the inhalation is complete, switch the gaze and awareness to the left eye, and begin exhalation through the left nostril, descending from the top of the nostril towards the tip of the nostril. The exhalation is complete at the tip of the left nostril. This is one round. The next round starts from the left nostril as mentioned above.

How Long

Do it for as long as you are comfortable with it. The breathing should be slow and deep, and if the breathing changes allow yourself to return to normal breathing when necessary. Stop the exercise if you experience any discomfort. Do not rush into switching the nostrils. It is better to stop the exercise if the breathing gets faster rather than moving the eyes and switching the nostrils faster.

Tips and Variations

This is a mind practice rather than a breathing practice per se. So do not worry if you happen to notice that the air escapes or enters through both nostrils during the exercise. As long as you are aware of one nostril versus the other that is engaged you are fine. Once you are comfortable with the practice, you can try it with your eyes opened. Another variation could be that you could try brief breath holds in between inhalations and exhalations. As this is kind of mental practice, the length for breath-holding need not necessarily be strict. You can allow the air to flow at its own pace, and be blocked in its own way.

Sadhura Moochu (Square Breathing)

प्रच्छर्दनविधारणाभ्यां वा प्राणस्य ॥३४॥

pracchardana-vidhāraṇa-ābhyāṁ vā prāṇasya

The inhalation, exhalation and retention all can be regulated in Pranayama as the Patanjali's Yoga Sutra teaches.

Pranayama is very forgiving, and it encourages you to experiment when it comes to patterns and durations. One of the ways we can easily alter different phases of inhalation, exhalation, and retention is to practice the equal phases of each step. That is what is described in this exercise.

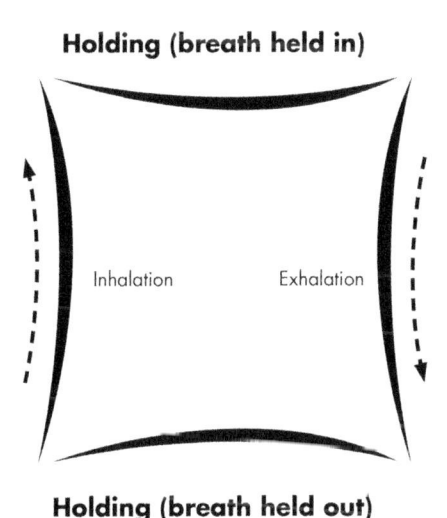

Holding (breath held in)

Inhalation   Exhalation

Holding (breath held out)

How To

All the breathing steps are through both nostrils, and therefore this is a good fit for anywhere you would not want to use the hands to perform the exercise. Use a chant of your choice that you will repeat during all the breathing/retention steps. Try your best to chant at the same pace all throughout the steps so they are somewhat equal. To begin the exercise, completely breathe out through both nostrils. 1) At the end of exhalation, hold the breath out for a comfortable number of counts, say three chants of Om Namasivaya, or any of your favorite chants. Remember that the chant is within your mind, not out loud. 2) At the end of three counts, begin inhaling for a total length of three chants. In other words, by the time you finish the third chant, you would have completed the complete inhalation. 3) Next, hold the breath for three counts of the chanting, and 4) Exhale for the length of three chants. This completes one round. At the end of exhalation, you can take a brief rest if needed or continue with the next round.

How Long

This exercise can be done for a period of 5–15 minutes. The total duration and the timing for each step of the exercise can be adjusted based on your comfort level.

Tips and Variations

Imagine a square! That is how you will be inhaling, holding in, exhaling and holding out. Every time you make it through all the corners it is kind of a home run! You could enjoy some relaxation at this point by watching the breath at your favorite location. Holding the breath out is a challenge in this exercise. It is always a good idea to start with low numbers all throughout the cycle such as three or four and then to slowly increase. I would suggest that any small variation in the length is normal and one does not have to worry about this being a major deviation. However, with practice one can gain control over the timing.

Sundara Chakra Pranayama

Chakras, the executive nexus
All along the spine
Keep them healthy
With a new combo trick

In this exercise, I have combined the traditional practice of meditating on the chakras with Pranayama and muscle movements and awareness and named it Sundara Chakra Pranayama. It is not only a part of my name but it was my grandfather's name as well, and most importantly, it refers to Sundarananda, a Siddhar some people think is the original name of Saint Thirumoolar. This exercise teaches us how we can use the breath along with awareness and muscular contractions to activate the seven chakras, which could be related to the nerve plexus along the spine. As this exercise requires the basic understanding of the chakra locations I provide a brief summary of the chakras:

1. **Mooladharam (root chakra).** This refers to an area surrounding the tail end of the spine and the coccygeal plexus. The movement of muscles in this region, the sphincter muscles around the rectum and the anus could potentially exercise this plexus. Mooladhara chakra has a prominent place as this is the basis for the formation of all other upper chakras according to the Yoga texts.

2. **Swadhittanam (pelvic chakra)** is located just above the Mooladharam. Swadhittanam is considered one of the areas that control both genital and urinary activities. This area can be exercised through voluntarily contracting the muscles associated with the genito-urinary contractions.

3. **Manipurakam (solar plexus).** This chakra is in the abdominal area around the navel and it can be exercised through the actions of tucking in or bulging out the tummy.

4. **Anahatham (heart chakra).** This is largely known as the heart center and it involves both the cardiac and pulmonary plexus. This chakra can be activated by the relaxation and contraction movements of the rib cage.

5. **Visuthi (throat chakra).** This is in the throat area and covers the pharyngeal plexus. This chakra can be activated by the movement of the neck as well by exercising the internal throat muscles via vocalization.

6. **Agna chakra (middle of the forehead).** This is normally referred to as the third eye and it is part of the carotid plexus. This chakra can be exercised through the movement of muscles in the forehead (in a frowning action) and through the movement of other facial muscles.

7. **Sahasrathalam (crown chakra).** This is the topmost part of the head and shares parts of the carotid plexus and it can be activated by raising the eyebrows which will cause an upward movement of the forehead muscles, as well as the scalp muscles.

This basic information will be helpful when you do this exercise as given below.

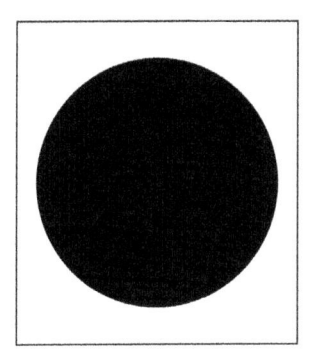

Common theme for Yeral

1. Inhale and hold the breath in
2. Contract the muscles around the Chakra point (see text for specific muscles)
3. Exhale and relax with normal breathing
4. Go to step 1 to repeat

Do this for all Chakras starting from Mooladharam, and moving up all the way to Sahasrathalam.

How To

Before starting the exercise decide if you want to do the exercise for all the chakras or if you just want to focus on one or a few because doing all the chakras in ascending (Yeral) and descending (Irangal) order will take at least an hour. Focusing on just one chakra completely can be done in about 10–15 minutes. So I want you to make sure you have enough time to complete this exercise before starting. This exercise is done in a seated pose that is comfortable to you and with closed eyes. Hands can be in Gnana mudra, or together on the lap or in any comfortable position. It is perfectly fine to move the body, or open the eyes, or relax the hands in between the exercise rounds. Also, please be aware of any injury or surgery to the areas you will be working on and avoid any extensive movements in those areas. Stop the exercise if any pain arises during the exercise.

There are two directions for this exercise: one is called the Yeral (ascending) that starts from the lowermost chakra (Mooladharam) to the uppermost chakra (Sahasrathalam). The other one is Irangal (descending) which is exactly the same route but in the opposite direction, starting from the crown and ending at the root. In both directions, each chakra is exercised for three rounds, with sufficient intermittent relaxation with awareness to the specific chakra being exercised. Let us see the steps for both ways individually:

Yeral (ascending):

The general pattern for the following seven steps of this exercise is: 1) Exhale through the nostrils completely. 2) Inhale through the nostrils and hold the breath. 3) Contract the muscle groups near the chakra repeatedly for as long as you can hold the breath. 4) Exhale through the nostrils. 5) Relax if necessary or repeat the cycle for a total of three times. 6) Relax. Breathe normally with your awareness on the specific chakra.

1. **Mooladharam:** Exhale through both nostrils, and take a deep breath for a completely full inhalation. Once the inhalation is complete, hold the breath. Bring your awareness to the root chakra, focusing on the tailbone area. Begin tightening the anal/rectal area by contracting the sphincter muscles, and once it is tightened to the fullest extent, relax it. You are not exhaling yet. Repeat the tightening and relaxation several times for as long as you can hold the breath. Once you have reached your maximum breath-holding capacity, then release the breath, and finish the contraction of the chakra also. If you would like to take a few breaths to relax, you can do it with complete awareness of the chakra. If not, continue with

the exercise by beginning the next round of inhalation. Once you finish three rounds of the exercise you can take a brief relaxation with chakra awareness.

2. **Swadhittanam:** Exhale completely. Inhale fully and hold. Contract the genito-urinary organs similar to holding the urination and then relax. Repeat this several times while holding the breath. At the end of breath-holding to your maximum capacity, exhale and then complete the contractions. Then relax with a few normal breaths or repeat the exercise for a total of three cycles. At the end of three cycles, relax while breathing normally and focusing your awareness on the chakra.

3. **Manipurakam:** Exhale completely, then inhale fully and hold. Move the tummy outwards as if it is bulging while holding the breath. The contracting action starts from the navel area. The tummy may already be full because of inhalation, but the bulging action will push the tummy out even more. Repeat the contractions as many times as possible while holding the breath. And then finally exhale and stop the contractions. Repeat this three more times relaxing in between rounds if necessary. At the end of three cycles, relax by breathing normally while focusing your awareness on the Manipurakam.

4. **Anahatham:** Exhale completely, inhale fully and hold the breath. Push the shoulder blades wide and then backward. This will create a gentle expansion of the chest. Imagine that the ribs and sternum are opening up from the inside. Repeat this kind of contraction and relaxation for as long as you can hold the breath. At the end of the breath holding, exhale and complete the contractions. Repeat this for a total of three cycles with intermittent rest if needed. Relax with normal breathing with awareness to the heart chakra.

5. **Visuthi:** Exhale completely, then inhale fully and hold the breath. Move the neck back as if the spine and the neck bone are aligned straight, something like a soldier. And then relax the neck by bringing it forward to its normal position. Repeat this neck movement several times for as long as you can hold the breath. At the end of the breath-holding exhale and complete the neck movements. Repeat this for a total of three cycles with intermittent rest if needed. Relax with normal breathing while bringing your awareness on the heart chakra.

6. **Agna:** Exhale completely, inhale fully and hold the breath. Contract the muscles in the forehead with a frowning action, and relax. Repeat this frowning action while holding the breath. At the end of the breath-holding, exhale and stop frowning. Repeat this for a total of three cycles with intermittent rest if needed. Relax with normal breathing with awareness on the Agna chakra.

7. **Sahasrathalam:** Exhale completely, then inhale fully and hold the breath. Raise the eyebrows slowly with awareness to the scalp and notice how the muscles on the head move toward each other. You might feel that the skin on the scalp all around the head moves towards the top of the head during this contraction. Relax by releasing the eyebrows. Repeat the contractions several times for as long as you can hold the breath. At the end of the breath-holding exhale and complete the eyebrow movements. Repeat this for a total of three cycles with intermittent rest if needed. Relax with normal breathing with awareness to the crown chakra.

At the end of the complete ascending series, you can finish the exercise for the day, or you can continue with the descending series.

Irangal (descending):

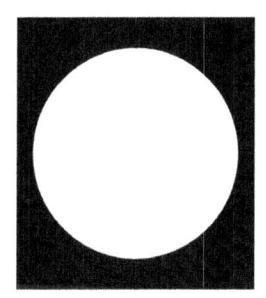

Common theme for Irangal

1. Exhale and hold the breath out
2. Contract the muscles around the Chakra point (see text for specific muscles)
3. Inhale and relax with normal breathing
4. Go to step 1 to repeat

Do this for all Chakras starting from Sahasrathalam, and moving down all the way to Mooladharam.

The Irangal series starts from the crown chakra and moves downwards to end at the root chakra. For the descending series the general pattern is as follows: 1) Through the nostrils, inhale fully filling the tummy, the lower ribs, and upper chest, and exhale completely by tucking the tummy in. 2) Hold the breath outside (external breath retention). 3) Contract the muscles associated with the chakra points several times for as long as you could hold the breath out. 4) Stop the contractions. 5) Inhale slowly through the nostrils. 6) Relax with a few normal breaths if needed. 7) Repeat steps 1–6 above for a total of 3 times, and 8) Breathe normally with awareness to the chakra and relax. While the muscles contractions are similar to the ascending series for most chakras, there is a variation for 2 chakras (heart and navel chakras), and please pay close attention to those below:

1. **Sahasrathalam:** Breathe in fully, then breathe out completely through the nostrils. Hold the breath out. Bring your awareness to the crown chakra. Raise the eyebrows several times as in the ascending series for as long as the breath can be held out. Once you are ready to breathe in finish the contractions and take a slow breath in. Take a few normal breaths. Repeat the cycle for a total of three times. At the end of three cycles perform normal breathing with awareness to the crown chakra.

2. **Agna:** Breathe in fully, and breathe out completely through the nostrils. Hold the breath out. Bring awareness to the middle of the forehead. Perform the frowning action several times as in the ascending series for as long as the breath can be held out. Once you are ready to breathe in, finish the contractions, and take a slow breath in. Take a few normal breaths. Repeat the cycle for a total of three times. At the end of three cycles return to normal breathing with your awareness on the Agna chakra.

3. **Visuthi:** Breathe in fully, then breathe out completely through the nostrils. Hold the breath out. Bring awareness to the throat chakra. Move the neck back like a soldier to align it almost to the spine, and then relax to bring it forward. Repeat this many times for as long as the breath can be held out. Once you are ready to breathe in finish the neck movements and take a slow breath in. Take a few normal breaths. Repeat the cycle for a total of three times. At the end of three cycles return to normal breathing with awareness on the throat chakra.

4. **Anahatham:** As mentioned above, the muscle contractions for this exercise are different from the ascending series. So pay close attention to the details of contractions. Breathe in fully, and breathe out completely through the nostrils. Hold the breath out. Bring awareness to the heart chakra. Cling the palms together, and bring the shoulder blades forward and closer to each other. This forms a slight inward curvature of the chest by pushing the middle

of the chest inwards. Remember, in the ascending series you would be doing this as an outward movement with the breath held in. On the contrary, here you are holding the breath out and curving the chest inwards. Use the movements of the shoulders to support this contraction. With the breath fully exhaled and then held, relax the shoulders and bring the chest to a normal level. Repeat this type of movement of the chest many times for as long as the breath can be held out. Once you are ready to breathe in, finish the contractions, and take a slow breath in. Take a few normal breaths. Repeat the cycle for a total of three times. At the end of three cycles perform normal breathing with awareness to the heart chakra.

5. **Manipurakam:** Again, this is another chakra where the contractions are different from the ascending series. Breathe in fully, and breathe out completely through the nostrils. Make sure the tummy is tucked in. Hold the breath out. Bring awareness to the navel area. Relax the tummy, and then tuck it in while holding the breath out. Pay close attention to the inward pulling of the tummy as if the navel is moving close to the spine. Repeat this many times for as long as the breath can be held out. Once you are ready to breathe in, finish the contractions, and take a slow breath in. Take a few normal breaths. Repeat the cycle for a total of three times. At the end of three cycles perform normal breathing with awareness to the navel chakra.

6. **Swadhittanam:** Breathe in fully, then breathe out completely through the nostrils. Hold the breath out. Bring awareness to the pelvic area. Perform the contractions of the genito-urinary organs similar to the ascending series, however by holding the breath out. Repeat this many times for as long as the breath can be held out. Once you are ready to breathe in, finish the contractions, and take a slow breath in. Take a few normal breaths. Repeat the cycle for a total of three times. At the end of three cycles perform normal breathing with awareness to the Swadhittana chakra.

7. **Mooladharam:** Breathe in fully, then breathe out completely through the nostrils. Hold the breath out. Bring awareness to the Mooladhara chakra, to the area around the tailbone and anal/rectal area. Perform the contractions of the anal/rectal area by repeatedly tightening and relaxing the sphincter muscles similar to the ascending series. Repeat this many times for as long as the breath can be held out. Once you are ready to breathe in, finish the neck movements, and take a slow breath in. Take a few normal breaths. Repeat the cycle for a total of three times. At the end of three cycles return to normal breathing with awareness on the Mooladhara chakra.

Once all the chakras are complete you can relax by breathing normally and focusing your awareness on the breath. Meditation is another option at the end of this exercise.

Tips and Variations

Finding the time to complete all of the above exercises in one session may not be practical for many of us. However, having seven chakras and seven days in a week makes it possible for an easy arrangement. I suggest practicing one chakra each day with both the ascending and descending exercise for that chakra. For example, for Sunday start with Mooladhara chakra. Perform the ascending first and then practice the descending for Mooladhara. All can be done within 15 minutes. Then work on other chakras, focusing on one every day. This might provide an opportunity to exercise all of them throughout the week. Awareness of the chakra during all stages of the practice is the key to a successful practice session. You might feel an excited state with a lot of energy and happiness for several hours when you do this exercise. Enjoy!

32

Karuvur Sithar Pranayama

Rule over the breath
Like a true master
Then follow, it will
Take you to the leader

This exercise floats within the Siddhar community as many have said about this in subtle ways. However, it was only when I was reading Karuvur Sithar's poem, that the technique for this exercise occurred to me. So I have named this exercise in his honor. This technique involves an inhalation, breath-holding and an exhalation. We use both nostrils. There is no timing for any of the phases, but it can be equal. There is a movement of throat muscles (laryngeal) during all three phases. It involves Ujjayi breathing (see Chapter 14). It also involves the internal recital of three chants: Vang, Ang, Sing. Explaining and learning this exercise is not easy, even with a video, unless you learn from the teacher in person. Let us try our best here.

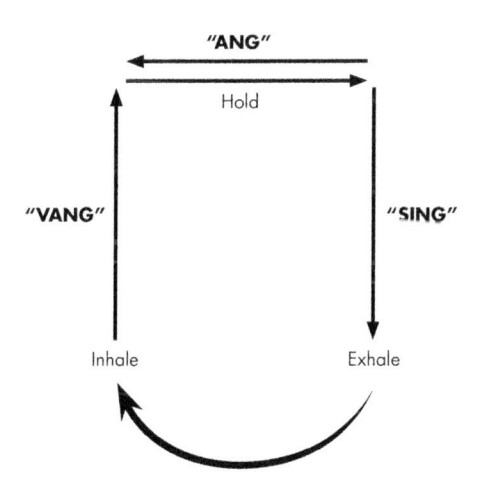

"ANG"
Hold

"VANG"   "SING"

Inhale   Exhale

How To

Before assembling the complete exercise, let us learn the bits and pieces of the exercise separately. Do not move to the next step if you are not thorough with learning the current step.

Ujjayi: To begin the exercise, practice the Ujjayi breathing for a few minutes.

Ng, ng, ng: Once the breathing is stabilized, then continue Ujjayi breathing by moving the tongue saying ng, ng, ng repeatedly (this is like saying the "ing" without much stress on the "i"). When you say ng, ng, ng repeatedly you will find that the tongue pulls inwards towards the throat. This retraction of the tongue is the main action during the inhalation, holding, and exhalation steps.

Vang: Once you are comfortable saying ng several times, learn to say Vang without pronouncing the V. The sound of V and the Vang should be in the mind; but the throat and tongue should be engaged as if you are saying the word Vang. The ng part of the Vang is the time at which there is a sustained Ujjayi sound during inhalation. Vang is the sound you would need to use for inhalation in this exercise.

Ang: The movement of the tongue in the Ang chanting phase is used to hold the breath at the level of the throat as if the back of the tongue is functioning like a cork to hold the breath. This Ang closure will happen after inhalation in the exercise.

Sing: This is used for the exhalation phase. Similar to the Vang pronunciation above, there is no opening of the mouth. Rather the tongue moves as if we say "Sing". The final part of ng in the Sing is the long sustained Ujjayi exhalation.

Now let us see how to assemble the above parts to do the Karuvur Sithar Pranayama:

1. **Inhalation:** Begin by Ujjayi breathing for a few minutes. Then inhale by saying Vang (again, you are not chanting aloud; you will

chant this in your mind but with the movement of the tongue only) along with the Ujjayi breathing. Keep inhaling as long as you can.

2. **Breath-hold:** Once the inhalation is complete, release the tongue from the Vang position, and move the tongue as if you are saying Ang while closing the throat with the back of the tongue as explained above. When you move the tongue to say Ang, during the A part, it is the movement to release the tongue from the previous position, and the ng part is to place it on the throat to seal the breath for holding. Thus ng in this phase is not Ujjayi breathing, rather it is the quiet breath-holding closure.

3. **Exhalation:** In the above breath-holding step, continue to hold for as long as you are comfortable. When you are ready to exhale, release the tongue from the Ang position, and move the tongue as if to pronounce the word Sing, without opening the mouth. After saying the first 2 letters "Si" then the tongue sits back in the ng position at the back of the throat to produce a sustained Ujjayi breathing sound. Exhale completely.

After the exhalation, go to the first step and repeat the exercise.

How Long

This is a powerful exercise for the throat chakra and can be done whenever you need more energy at the throat, perhaps you will find this useful before a meeting or a lecture. The best thing is that you do not have to use the hands for breath-holding, and therefore can easily do this anywhere in a sitting posture. The duration could be from 5–15 minutes. Longer practice might make your tongue muscles get tired or it may cause you pain. Also, at the beginning stages, a tingling feeling in the throat might make you cough or discourage you from doing the practice. You can overcome this with practice.

Tips and Variations

Karuvur Sithar Pranayama requires some imagination to move the tongue as if you are pronouncing the chant, but without the sound of the chant, and without opening the mouth. During the initial stages practice a lot of Ujjayi with just the tongue movement like you say ng, ng, ng repeatedly. This will help you to move into the practice quickly. If you do not understand how I explained it here, ask someone who understood it. Also, keep the inhalation, breath-hold, and exhalation steps shorter during the learning phase so you will not have to overstrain on too many things at once. Always build it up slowly with a lot of awareness to the area you are working with, as well as the breath, and the mind.

33

Karai Moochu (Crying Breathing)

நானே பொய்
என் நெஞ்சும் பொய்
என் அன்பும் பொய், ஆனால்
வினையேன் அழுதால் உன்னைப் பெறலாமே

— திருவாசகம், மாணிக்கவாசகர்

I am falsehood

My heart is a myth

My love is a deceit

But if I cry I can get you (Lord)

– Manickavasakar in Thiruvasakam

The word Karai in Tamil means to cry. It has other meanings like call, dissolve, and boundary of a water body (like an ocean, river, dam, pond, etc.). Lots of literary works from the ancient Saiva tradition and the Siddha tradition talk about the importance of crying, especially by way of self-criticism for not crying. Manickavasagar says, "கசிந்துருகேன்... கரைந்திடிலேன்... முட்டிலேன், தகலகிறேன்..." Which translates as "I am such a stone hearted person that I do not cry, dissolve myself (heart)". While crying is generally considered a sign of weakness, there are a lot of physiological, emotional, and social benefits of crying. Crying is known to stimulate several neuromodulators, as well as other factors that would reduce pain, improve mood, cardiovascular functions, and energy status, and overall emotional wellbeing. As per the Tamil definition, this exercise could dissolve the pain, anxiety, suppressed emotions, and accumulated toxins, and it can serve as a boundary to float our emotions up and down but without breaking them.

In this exercise, we mimic just one of the several characteristics of the actual crying process – the breathing. This exercise will use gentle repetitive breathing in and out similar to quietly sobbing.

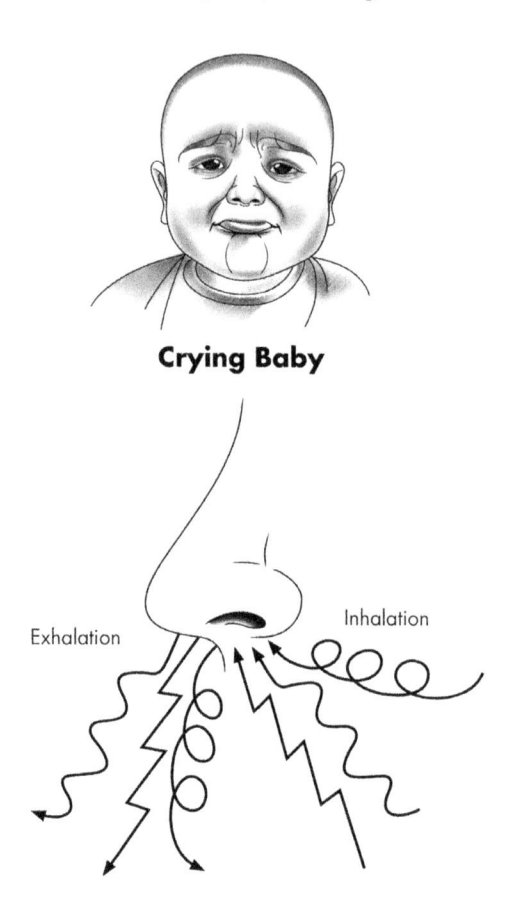

Crying Baby

Exhalation

Inhalation

How To

We will be bringing awareness to the following areas and using these techniques:

Annakku: Become aware of the naso/oropharyngeal region. It is the area of the soft palate and the areas coming from the nasal passage. If you move the tip of your tongue along the hard palate and reach the soft palate that is the area you will be focusing on.

Modified Ujjayi: We will use a variation of Ujjayi breathing for this exercise. Ujjayi is discussed in Chapter 14 of this book. However, the variation we will use here is that it is not the single smooth inhalation/exhalation. Rather it is the fractionated inhalation and exhalation. That is, the inhalation is split into several small steps of continuous inhalation. Similarly, the exhalation is fractionated into several steps as well. There is no counting the number of steps up or down.

Now we are ready with the tools. Let's go to the practice!

Close your eyes, let your gaze within your closed eyes be at the middle of the forehead or at the crown chakra. Then bring your awareness to the Annakku. Start the inhalation by several steps of Ujjayi as mentioned above. The inhalation happens in several steps, and each step is sensed at the soft palate. Once you are completely done with the inhalation, then begin the exhalation in the same manner of repeating the Ujjayi breathing in several steps. What you will find is that the exhalation steps will make the air hit the nasopharyngeal area repeatedly. You will have a strong stimulation of the Agna chakra, a sensation you can feel in the middle of the forehead. This is associated with the stimulation of olfactory lobe neurons, and strong stimulation of salivary and lacrimal glands. At the end of exhalation, you could take a break by taking a few normal breaths or continue with the next round of inhalation.

How Long

You do not have to partake in this practice for an extended amount of time. Crying for a long time will drain our energy and can cause negative physical and psychological effects including depression. It is better to keep this for 3–5 rounds with about three minutes of watching the breathing at the Agna center in between the rounds. You could try this once in the morning, noon, evening, and before going to bed. Doing it just before bedtime might be a good way to clear the emotions, cleanse the eyes, and irrigating the nasal and oral passages with healing biomolecules. Always be cautious to avoid becoming overwhelmed by emotions that have been suppressed for too long. Practice control and do it slowly in a stepwise manner. This is, after all, an exercise about boundaries!

Tips and Variations

If you cannot stop, do not start this exercise in public. In some individuals, crying can stimulate the reappearance of previously suppressed emotions. Practice caution when approaching this exercise as too much could make you worse than how you were when you started the exercise. To avoid any negative outcomes of the exercise, my suggestion would be to use a subject or theme on which you want to cry: for example, your favorite natural scenery, the open sky, or the name of your favorite deity. That will keep people and related emotions at a safe distance. When you have a good handle on the exercise and the emotions, you can revisit those suppressed emotions slowly, one at a time. The goal of this exercise is to dissolve everything that is bothering us, to cleanse us, and to make us clear and happy—a factory reset!

34

Kottavi Moochu (Yawning Breathing)

கூண்டுவிழுஞ் சீவன் மெள்ளக் கொட்டாவி கொண்டாற்போல்
மாண்டுவிழு முன்னேநான் மாண்டிருப்ப தெக்காலம்.

As one yawns before going to bed
When will my ego die before my life ends

— **Pathiragiriyar Sithar**

If you happen to yawn reading this Chapter, it is not because this book is boring, but in fact, this Chapter is on yawning! Kottu in Tamil language means to dump something, usually in large quantities. Avi means steam, air, vapor, or life. Kottavi means yawning in Tamil. The name suggests it is a way to dump a large quantity of air into your system. When do we yawn? When bored, in cold conditions, stressful situations, and when feeling empathetic. My grandmother (Appayee) yawns whenever she calls out deity names during every one of her prayers. Athletes are seen yawning before competitions. Yawning is spontaneous, or social when it is spread from others. Studies suggest it might cool the brain, improve the blood circulation to the brain, cerebrospinal fluid circulation and the intake of the large volume of air increases heart rate, reduces blood pressure, and overall looks like it is preparing us to get active. That makes sense when it is social, as in our animal kingdom when one yawns based on the current situation or stress, others will yawn, and as a result, the whole group gets energized and becomes ready for any threat to the group. This is the way to quickly increase the energy level of a group, and therefore for competitive teams, yawning all together might be a good thing to do before a game. It will also stimulate salivation, and as always, the associated good stuff in it. The name kottavi referring to dumping a large volume of air into the system seems to make sense. As per Pathiragiriyar, it is the acceptance of kottavi, which means receiving, taking in a large quantity of air. It is not so much about exhalation. In that poem, he refers to how we get a lot of air before going to bed. Maybe that is a way to energize ourselves, providing a good amount of oxygen as all the organ systems will be resting; it is like eating before going to bed so you will not be awakened by your hunger. If you are already energetic there is no need for external input, however, yawning happens whenever the body feels a deficiency, and it makes one alert.

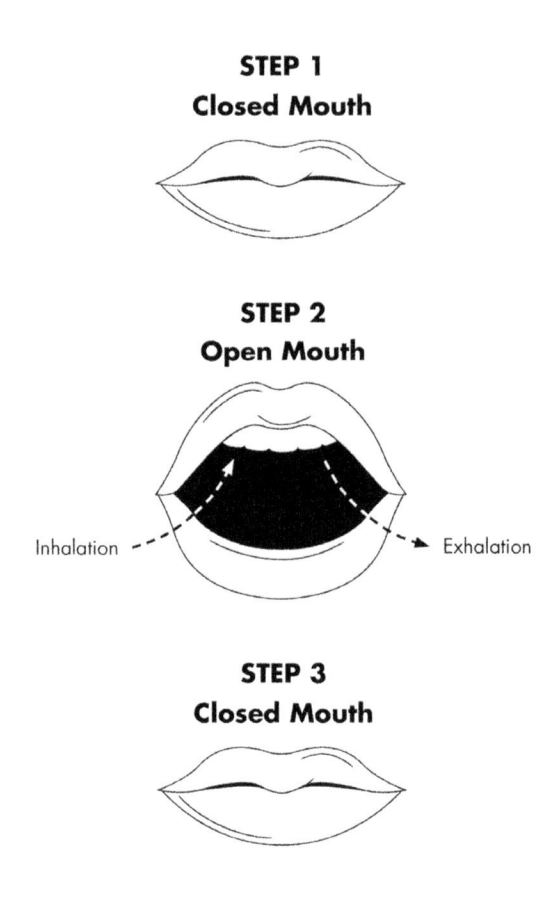

STEP 1
Closed Mouth

STEP 2
Open Mouth

Inhalation — Exhalation

STEP 3
Closed Mouth

How To

No explanations are necessary for yawning! However, there are a few additional points. Let the inhalations focus on the soft palate area. Do not rush in the inhalation/exhalation cycle; you might hyperventilate. Inhale slowly, as you would normally yawn. Maybe you could use some Ujjayi type of control on the inhalation so it is smooth and long. Open the jaws as much as you can during the inhalation to reach the maximum at complete inhalation. Once the inhalation is complete, begin to breathe out through the mouth. Keep the exhalations as slow as possible through the mouth. Keep closing the jaws as you proceed with the exhalation. Towards the end of exhalation, when the mouth is completely closed, exhalation still continues through the nostrils to the fullest degree. You could watch the breath with awareness to any of the upper chakras. I prefer the crown chakra because of the possible stimulation of all the nerves in the scalp. And, remember my grandmother yawned at every prayer. I think that might have been her way of communicating with the sky through her crown chakra. After the brief relaxation, you can repeat the yawning a few more times.

How Long

Do this exercise whenever you need more energy instantly. You can repeat this for up to 15 times with intermittent resting breaths so you will not hyperventilate. Practice caution and be watchful of how you feel physically and emotionally. You can do this during any transition during the day. It might be better to take a small break to use the restroom, or water breaks every 90 minutes or so during our workday. During those short transitions, you could try this to renew energy before returning to your work.

Tips and Variations

Cover your mouth to avoid any dust, pollutants, or germs entering, or if you would like to keep it private, i.e., not spreading the yawning to others around you. During a classroom activity, you are teaching, if you see a little boredom, you could ask the class to do this a few times to stimulate energy, giggles and renewed focus. If you are a student and your teacher does not have a clue about this Pranayama, see the first tip above.

One variation could be exhaling through the nostrils. It might have a different effect on the overall body temperature, but it is not well studied. Be aware of your breath and the response within your physical and emotional systems.

Thantha Moochu (Tooth Breathing)

Strong like ivory

But suffers a little dent

Burns the pain

With the power of breath

Thantham means tooth or ivory in Tamil. This Pranayama can be an instant pain reliever if there is any acute toothache due to trapped particles, or sensitive nerves. This is based on my experience. My observation was that the tongue stretch, as in the case of lifting the tongue to touch the soft palate and touching it just with the tip, and bringing awareness to the tip of the tongue would make the tip of the tongue burning hot. This could be due to the activation of stretch-induced receptor activation like the ones stimulated by the chili pepper (called the TRPV receptors). This activation is kind of contagious, in the sense that it does not stop at the tongue, or the place it touches, but spreads possibly through neurons to other areas where the contacting neurons travel. It is like spreading capsaicin using the tip of the tongue as an applicator. I used this technique one day when I got something stuck in my gum. It was bothering me despite repeated flossing and using tooth powders like Dhanthathavana churnam, or Tripala churnam. It made me think that I needed something hot in the gum. Then this tongue tip burning fact occurred to me, and I tried to test it. It worked! Within a few minutes, the pain went away. I wanted to share this with you and see if it works for your toothache too, at least for minor ones. Do please let me know if it works for chronic toothaches.

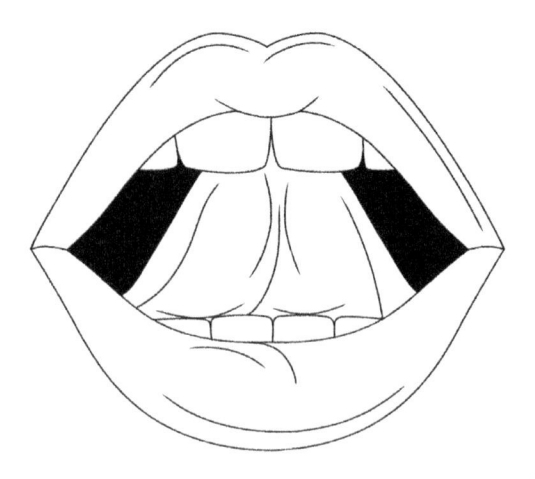

How To

Move the tip of the tongue to the area of the gum that is experiencing the pain. Make sure that only the tip of the tongue, not the whole or middle part, touches the gum. You will notice that the tongue muscle has tonicity that will allow you to experience several connects and disconnects between the tip of the tongue and the gum, which is normal. Breathe slowly through the nostrils with awareness to the area of pain. Imagine the breath originates and returns to the same area as you inhale and exhale. Try to take long breaths. But the major awareness is at the top of the tongue and the area of the gum. Within a few minutes or a few breaths, you might feel the burning sensation spreading from the tip of the tongue into the gum. Once in the gum, it will slowly diffuse into the painful areas too. As the burning sensation travels into the pain area, it makes the pain go away, just like what capsaicin would do in that area. Continue to do the exercise until the pain subsides.

How Long

You could do this exercise until you see a reduction in pain. However, one limiting factor could be the pain that could arise in the tongue itself due to prolonged stretching. You could take a break by releasing the tongue and doing some normal breathing and then do the exercise for a few more minutes. There is no specific number of times I would suggest for this exercise, but one can do it for as long as there is no discomfort, and until the pain goes away.

Tips and Variations

Be completely aware of the pain, the area of the pain, and the breath. Do it only to reduce the pain because the other effects of this exercise on the brain's function are not known. There is a variation of this exercise which is called the Kechari mudra where the tip of the tongue is placed at the soft palate. This exercise can be combined with Ujjayi breathing or done with normal deep breathing.

Kireeda Moochu (Crown Chakra Churn Pranayama)

Churn the chakra with the breath
Move up the ladder of consciousness
Open up the doors to the heavens
Get closer to the Oneness, every breath

The crown chakra is an important part of connecting our consciousness with the Vignanamaya Kosha or to an elevated state of consciousness. For that one needs to be aware of the crown chakra and let the nerves in those areas become responsive to our breathing, and mindfulness regulations. This exercise could help us improve our awareness of the crown chakra.

How To

Breathe in and out normally with awareness to the crown chakra for a few minutes. Once you are able to feel/sense the crown chakra as you breathe, slowly begin breathing in and out of the crown chakra. This further improves the awareness of the crown chakra. Continue this breath awareness for a few minutes. Once you are able to connect the breath and mind with the crown chakra, then you can begin raising the eyebrows several times as you breathe in. The inhalation is divided into several fractions. There is no specific number for these fractions or steps. However, each fraction is synchronized with a contraction (raising and releasing the eyebrow). This allows multiple contractions during inhalation, and can quickly improve your awareness of the crown chakra. Once the inhalation is over, stop the contractions, and exhale slowly through the nostrils. At the end of the exhalation, you can rest with awareness to the crown chakra or continue to the next round with a fresh inhalation and contraction.

CROWN CHAKRA

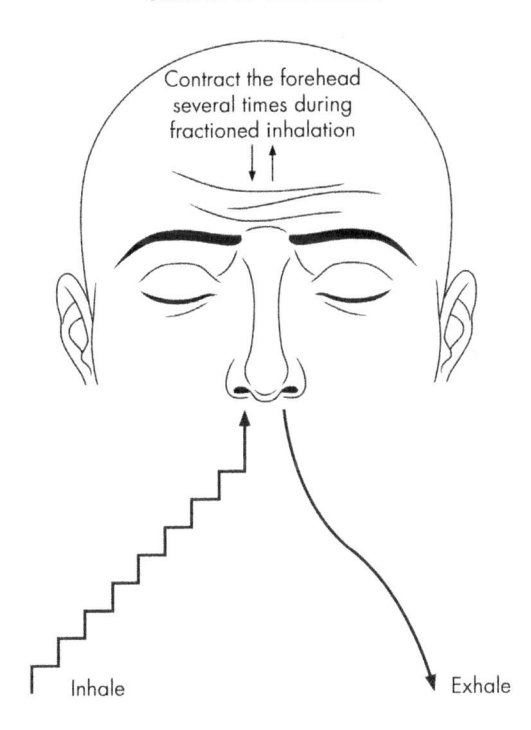

Contract the forehead several times during fractioned inhalation

Inhale   Exhale

How Long

You can do this for seven breaths/cycles with or without intermittent normal breath and watching of the crown chakra. After the seven cycles of contractions, you can meditate on the crown chakra with normal breathing for any length of time. Do this exercise whenever you would like to stimulate the topmost part.

Tips and Variations

As we saw in Chapter 31, the Sundara Chakra Pranayama is an effective way of activating all the chakras individually by combining the breathing. As that exercise is already long and complicated I have given this individual chakra exercise variation as a separate exercise. For the basic summary of chakras and the muscle contractions associated with individual chakra activation, please read Chapter 31 Sundara Chakra Pranayama.

37

166 Mathirai Moochu (166 Count Breathing)

நூறும் அறுபதும் ஆறும் வலம்வர
நூறும் அறுபதும் ஆறும் இடம்வர
நூறும் அறுபதும் ஆறும் எதிரிட
நூறும் அறுபதும் ஆறும் புகுவரே.

Noorum arubathum aarum valamvara

Noorum arubathum aarum idamvara

Noorum arubathum aarum edhirida

Noorum arubathum aarum puhuvare.

Hundred and sixty-six going around the right

Hundred and sixty-six going around the left

Hundred and sixty-six going against each other

One will reach one hundred and sixty-six

There are several methods from Thirumanthiram on how to do the Pranayama, and some of them were discussed in my earlier book PranaScience: Decoding Yoga Breathing. This one is also from Thirumanthiram, where the technique may not be new but the timing for the technique and the final outcome of the exercise are defined in this poem by Thirumoolar, the saint who wrote Thirumanthiram. Although there are several versions of the interpretation of this poem, the most common one that is accepted by several scholars is the version I am providing here. This exercise can be built up after prolonged practice. The main outcome of this exercise is that this will extend the life way beyond one hundred, another 60, and another 6. I think 166 might be the maximum number of years one could live in this body, and that lengthy lifetime can be achieved by this breathing exercise.

All steps of inhalation and exhalation are for a length of 166 mathirai (approximately 20 times of Om Namasivaya chanting for each step)

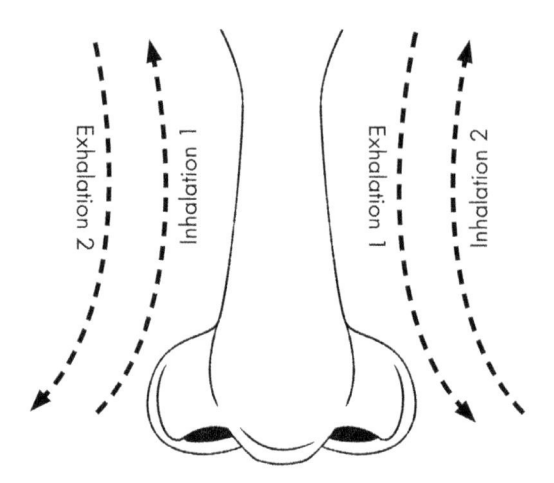

How To

First, perform long deep breathing (Dheerga Swasam) as prescribed in Chapter 1. Then continue with Alternate Nostril Breathing (Chapter 3). Each of the above exercises can be done for about 3–5 minutes. Once you complete both of them in that sequence, continue with the Alternate Nostril Breathing. This time you will be using a mantra that will help you to hold the breath for 166 mathirai. You know from Chapter 7 how to calculate mathirai. Use a chant and repeat it so you will be able to count 166 mathirai. The chant Om Namasivaya for 20 times would be approximately 160 mathirai; however adding the slight pauses, it could amount to 166 mathirai. That is the time for complete slow inhalation through the right nostril, and then the same 20 chants (166 mathirai) for exhalation through the left nostril. At the end, inhale through the left nostril, and then exhale through the right nostril, each step for 166 mathirai. This might appear to be a tough task. However, with practice, one might be able to master this length.

How Long

One could do this exercise for a period of 24 minutes each time, three times a day. If it is not possible to practice for a long time, then the practice time can be reduced to a comfortable level and can be slowly increased as one matures through the practice. Also, the time for each segment (inhalation, exhalation) can be reduced as per one's comfort level. Discontinue the exercise if there is an uneasy feeling in the mind or body.

Tips and Variations

Start from a low number, say 10 counts or less for each inhalation, and exhalation steps. Once you get comfortable, slowly increase one count every week. When you come to around 16, you can increase to the next level after 1–3 months of continuous practice.

Further Learning

1. PranaScience.com. Official website of Sundar Balasubramanian. This website contains learning materials including videos, published research articles, interviews, blog posts, and events.

2. Sundar Balasubramanian. PranaScience: Decoding Yoga Breathing. A book on Thirumoolar's Thirumanthiram with special emphasis to Pranayama. Notion Press, 2017.

3. http://anmolmehta.com/. Official website of Anmol Mehta, explaining various Asana, Kriya, Pranayama and Meditative techniques.

4. http://www.abundantwellbeing.com/. Official website of Nischala Joy Devi. Resourceful website to understand the power of Yoga in healing.

5. Sri Swami Satchidananda. The Breath of Life: Integral Yoga Pranayama: Step-by-Step Instructions in the Yogic Breathing Practices. Integral Yoga Publications, Yogaville, VA. 1976.

பின்னுரை

அன்புள்ள சுந்தருக்கு:

முழுவதும் படித்துவிட்டேன். உண்மையில் இது உன்னுடைய மேலான பங்களிப்புகளில் ஒன்றாக நிச்சயம் கருதப்படும். உண்மையில் இதை அழகாக எழுதியுள்ளாய். சின்ன, எளிமையான கவித்துவம் கூடிய வழிநடைச் செய்யுள் ஒரு அருமையான உத்தி. அதைத் தொடர்ந்த அறிமுகமும், படங்களும், குறிப்புகளும், படிப்பவரது கூடவே நடந்து அவரது கேள்வி எழும்தருணத்தில் அதைச் சொல்லுவது போல எழுதியிருக்கிறாய்.

இதை ஒருவர் தன்னுடைய வாழ்நாள் துணைவனாகக் கருதி ஆழ்ந்த, நிதானமான பயிற்சிக்குப் பயன்படுத்திக் கொள்ளலாம். பிறகு அவரவர்க்கு மிகவும் உகந்த பயிற்சிகளில் தோய்ந்து முழுமையும் இன்பமும் அடையலாம். சில புத்தகங்கள் ஒருமுறை மட்டும் வாசித்தலுக்கானவை அல்ல. அவைகள் ஒருவருடனே உறைந்து அவர் வளரும் தோறும் வளர்ந்து அவருள் கரையும் தன்மையன. அத்தகைய நூல் இது.

இதன் மூலம் ஒருவர் மூச்சை நம்பகமான ஒரு துணையாக, எக்காலத்தும் தன்னை அறியும் திருவுகோலாகக் காலப்போக்கில் ஆக்கிக்கொள்ளமுடியும். அப்பொழுது அவர் காலனை உதைக்கும் கலையறியப்பெறுவர் என்பது திண்ணம்.

குருவருளால் இது சித்தித்துள்ளது.

அன்புடன்
தங்கமணி

(முனைவர் தங்கமணி நித்யானந்தம் ஒரு இயற்கை வாழ்வியல் வல்லுனர், பறவை ஆர்வலர், புகைப்படக் கலைஞர், மற்றும் கரம்பக்குடி யோக அறக்கட்டளையின் நிறுவனர்).

Backword (English Translation)

Dear Sundar:

I just completed reading this. Truly this book will be considered as one of your best contributions. You have written it so beautifully. Short and simple poems at the beginning are a nice technique. It is followed by introductions, diagrams, and technical details that move with the reader; and whenever there is a question arising you have answered it there.

One can use this book as a lifelong guide to learn the practice. Then they can immerse in those practices to joy and perfection. Some books are not just for one time reading. Such books stay with them, grow with them, and dissolve in them. This is one such a book.

Through this book one can make the breathing as a reliable companion for ever, and also as a key to open the inner self. At that point s/he knows the technique of kicking the death.

This book is possible with the blessings of the Guru.

With love

Thangamani

(Dr. Thangamani Nithyanantham is an expert on Natural Living, birdwatching, photography, and the Founder of Yoga Arakkattalai, Karambakkudi, India)

Printed in Great Britain
by Amazon